THE NEW
LOVE AND SEX
AFTER 60

REVISED EDITION

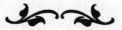

ROBERT N. BUTLER, M.D.
AND MYRNA I. LEWIS, Ph.D.

D0188487

BALLANTINE BOOKS · NEW YORK

A Ballantine Book
Published by The Ballantine Publishing Group

Copyright © 1976, 1988, 1993, 2002 by Robert N. Butler and
Myrna I. Lewis

Originally published by Harper & Row Publishers in 1976.
Revised editions published in 1988 by Harper & Row Publishers
and in 1993 by The Ballantine Publishing Group, a division of
Random House, Inc.

www.ballantinebooks.com

Library of Congress Card Number: 2001118401

ISBN 0-345-44211-3

Text design by Holly Johnson

Manufactured in the United States of America

Third Revised Edition: February 2002

10 9 8 7 6 5 4 3 2 1

THE NEW LOVE AND
SEX AFTER 60

CONTENTS

CONTENTS

PREFACE

We are in the midst of a longevity revolution. In the past century, Americans have gained an additional thirty years of life. This is more than has been achieved in the preceding five thousand years of human history! Increases in life expectancy in the industrialized world are continuing to grow and, with any luck, will spread to the developing world as well. But few have begun to absorb what this means in our personal lives. Many of us can now look forward to an additional twenty to thirty years of life after we reach sixty. We can expect to be in at least reasonably good health for much of that time—and health in later life continues to improve. What is needed now is a revolution in our thinking about what it means to be older. Attitudes toward love and sex are a good place to start!

Times have already changed since we wrote the first edition of *Love and Sex after Sixty* in 1976. A quarter of a century ago the subject made a lot of people uncomfortable—in fact, sex for older people was a taboo topic. Typical of this attitude, a major Florida newspaper refused to advertise our book's publication, declaring it "too prurient for the general public." When we appeared on network television in the late 1970s, the interviewer (now an older woman herself) warned parents to keep their teenagers and small children out of the room, away from the dangerous topic of late-life sexuality. Health professionals admitted that they rarely, if ever, discussed sexuality as part of their medical and psychological evaluation of older people. Physicians and other health-care workers had remarkably little training in human sexuality for any age group. The media treated the subject of sex after sixty with ridicule and disparagement— if they addressed it at all. And many older people themselves were unclear about the propriety of sexuality in the latter part of their lives.

In the face of all this negativity, how did we become involved in writing about love and sex after sixty? For years a number of older people had come to see us in our psychotherapy practices, insisting that their sexuality be taken seriously. They wanted advice on how to maintain relationships, whether old or new. They wanted help with physical problems that were interfering with sexual activity. They wanted their families, their doctors, and the world in general to recognize them as full, functioning adults. It dawned on us that they needed a book of their own on the vital topic of late-life sexuality.

Some twenty-five years have passed since then. The subject is no longer taboo. The sexuality of older people has become a generally accepted fact of life, helped along by public figures like Senator Robert Dole openly discussing his erectile problems (connected with prostate cancer) and his relief in being able to do something to resolve them. Great writers like Gabriel García Márquez in *Love in the Time of Cholera* have chosen the theme of late-life love. Even TV sitcoms now occasionally portray older persons conducting romances and maintaining relationships that plainly involve sexuality.

The baby boomers are an added driving force in liberating later-life sexuality, first as advocates for their parents and soon, as the oldest boomers approach sixty years of age, for themselves. Just as they led the sexual revolution for the young in the 1960s, it is only a matter of time before they notice the need for a wholesale transformation of the meaning of love and sexuality up to the very limits of life itself.

Our aim in this newest edition is to continue to bring people the latest data on the dynamic subject of sexuality as they grow older. Although easy access to reliable and up-to-date information on late-life sexuality still remains problematic, there is much that is new and heartening. The diagnosis and treatment of sexual problems continue to improve. As one example, the options for treating erectile dysfunction in older men have increased dramatically in the past few years, especially with the introduction of the little blue pill, Viagra. A dozen or so new medications are in various stages of clinical trials, waiting to enter the huge market now labeled "life enhancement" or "lifestyle" drugs.

Advances in treating male dysfunction are leading to a fresh focus on the sexuality of older women, underscored by a recognition that, because of their longer lives, women represent an even larger pharmaceutical consumer group than men. Market-driven and drug-oriented as these efforts are, they nevertheless hold the promise of serious scrutiny of a topic that previously attracted little research attention—namely the older female sexual response cycle. The phallocentric era of sexual research with a focus mainly on male erectile capacity is giving way to equal curiosity about women and the conditions that interfere with their sexual expression.

Rapid advances are also occurring in understanding menopause and its impact on the final third of women's lives. The huge Women's Health Initiative sponsored by the National Institutes of Health, the ongoing Boston-based Nurses' Health Study, and a wide variety of other public and private research efforts are beginning to provide valuable insights into options for insuring women's health after midlife.

Health professionals, the public, and older people themselves have also become more aware of the continuing importance of emotional relationships as we grow older. What roles do love and sex play in giving meaning to later life? How do you keep a romance going through fifty or more years of a relationship? How do you start all over again after divorce or your partner's death? What are the advantages older people bring to the art of love and life? What are the disadvantages? How do you manage problems? Whom do you turn to for information and advice? The ongoing desire for more information led us to the work of revising the material in this book once again. We hope we have supplied some of the answers in this latest edition.

On a final note, we want to emphasize again the extraordinary gift of life that we now have. How can we take full advantage of our added thirty years of life expectancy? One way is to recognize that love and sex after sixty is no longer a surprise. It is a fact of life.

An Internet Postscript: A rapidly growing number of persons over sixty (about 20 percent of those aged sixty to eighty) are on-line and able to use the Internet. Nonetheless, the majority still do not have this option. For this reason we have provided addresses and phone numbers rather than Web sites for resource materials listed in this text. Internet users can simply log on to any search engine (we personally love Google) for further information on the subjects and sources that we mention.

ACKNOWLEDGMENTS

The authors would like to thank the following people:

Barbara E. C. Paris, M.D., Clinical Associate Professor, Department of Geriatrics, the Mount Sinai School of Medicine, New York

S. Mitchell Harman, M.D., Ph.D., Director, Kronos Longevity Research Institute, Phoenix, Arizona

Panayiotis Tsitouras, M.D., Associate Professor, Department of Geriatrics, University of Arkansas, Little Rock, Arkansas

E. Douglas Whitehead, M.D., F.A.C.S., Associate Clinical Professor of Urology, Albert Einstein College of Medicine, New York, Director, Association for Male Sexual Dysfunction, Director, New York Phalloplasty

THE NEW LOVE AND
SEX AFTER 60

CHAPTER 1

❧ ❧

THE NEW LOVE AND SEX AFTER 60

The best authorities on whether love and sex can exist in later life are older people themselves. Frank and Marianne have been together forty-six years. They've led unremarkable lives in terms of success and lucky breaks and have had more than their share of tragedies. Yet in their late seventies they are enthusiastic, optimistic, *and in love*. Frank says of Marianne, "I love this woman more each day." Marianne replies, "I couldn't have asked for a better partner—he's kind, sweet, funny . . . he is everything a woman could want." Both are quick to add that it is their relationship that has been the core of their sense of satisfaction in life—and their sexual closeness is an indispensable part of their affection for each other. These two are not alone in their point of view. Any

1

of us who has worked professionally with older people (or is personally older) could cite scores of examples of similar attitudes among older persons, married or single.

Sound research data beyond the clinical observations of those working with older people is another story. The United States lacks a truly comprehensive national survey of sexuality that encompasses the older population. The available information includes the important but now outdated and limited Kinsey studies (first published in 1948), the physiologic investigations of Masters and Johnson, and the findings of both the Duke Longitudinal Studies and the Baltimore Longitudinal Study on Aging. Questionnaire surveys of self-reported sexual activity among older people have been conducted by mail (for example, by Consumers Union), but these provide information only on those who volunteer. Other studies have age cutoffs for their subjects, usually at sixty or seventy. The outcome is that essential facts and figures on the nature and frequency of sexual activity among older persons, including its association with marital and health status or any other variable in people's lives, are lacking.

One thing is certain, however. Our society is in the midst of an immense demographic change. Every day over six thousand Americans turn sixty. Altogether, forty-five million people or one out of every six of us are sixty or older. By the year 2006, baby boomers will begin to dramatically expand the ranks of the older population as they themselves start turning sixty. In about twenty five years, one in five Americans, including the boomers, will be over sixty-five—a historically unprecedented 20 percent of the population.

The definition of old age is changing. In June 2000, *The New Yorker Magazine* ran a cartoon showing a woman announcing to her husband, "Good news, honey—seventy is the new fifty." That same year a Harris Poll found that only 14 percent of respondents believed chronological age was the best marker of old age. Instead, 41 percent cited a "decline in physical ability"—a highly variable event—as the best evidence of the beginning of old age. According to this definition, people in good health are younger longer, whereas anyone who gets sick becomes older sooner. As for disability itself, studies show that there have been significant declines in disability rates since 1982. Heart disease and stroke alone have been reduced 60 percent since 1950.

In light of all this, what can we safely say about sexuality in later life? Our views on this topic have not yet caught up with the slowly changing character of aging. Many people—not only the young and middle-aged but older people themselves—are quite uniformly negative about the prospects of continued sexual interest and ability. Many simply assume that the game is over somewhere in late midlife or early later life. They couldn't be more wrong. In spite of the scarcity of nationwide data, we turn to our own clinical and research work and the work of other gerontologists and researchers to demonstrate that relatively healthy older people are often capable of enjoying sex—often until *very* late in life. Moreover, those who do have sexual problems can frequently be helped.

We have written this book for those older men and women who are presently or potentially interested in sexuality and would like to know more about what is likely to happen to their sexuality over time. We will offer solutions to sexual problems that may occur, and propose ways of countering the negative attitudes that older people may experience—within themselves, from family members, from the medical and psychotherapeutic professions, and from society at large. We especially want older people to know that their concerns and problems are not unique, that they are not alone in their experience, and that many others feel *exactly as they do*. Even those people who have had a lively enthusiasm and capacity for sex all their lives often need information, support, and sometimes various kinds of treatment in order to continue engaging in sexual activity as the years go by. In addition, people for whom sex may not have been especially satisfying in their younger days may find that it is now possible to improve the quality of the experience despite their long-standing difficulties.

Sex and sexuality are pleasurable, rewarding, and fulfilling experiences that can enhance the middle and later years. But they are also—as everyone knows—enormously complex psychologically. Every one of us carries with us throughout our lives a weight of attitudes related to sexuality that have been shaped by our genes, our parents, our families, our teachers, and our society, some of which are positive and some negative, some of which we realize and many of which we are unaware.

Because of this, it is useful to understand what underlies so many of the attitudes and problems about sex that one encounters. If you are an older person, be prepared for the likelihood of conflicting feelings within yourself and contradictory attitudes from the outside world. Should older people have sex lives? Are they even able to make love? Do they really want to? Is it appropriate—that is, "normal" or "decent"—or is sexual interest a sign of "senility" and brain disease (he/she has gone "daft"), poor judgment, or an embarrassing inability to adjust to aging with the proper restraint and resignation?

How much less troubling it would be to accept the folklore of cookie-baking grandmothers who bustle around the kitchen making goodies for their loved ones while rocking-chair grandfathers puff on their pipes and reminisce. Idealized folk figures like these are not supposed to have sex lives of their own. After all, they represent the parents and grandparents we all remember from our childhood, rather than fellow adults with the same needs and desires that we have.

As an older man or woman, you may find that love and sex in later life, when they are acknowledged at all, will be patronizingly thought of as "cute" or "sweet," like the puppy love of teenagers; but even more likely, they will be ridiculed, a subject for jokes that have undercurrents of disdain and apprehensiveness at the prospect of growing older. Our language is full of telltale phrases: older men become "dirty old men," "old fools," or "old goats" where sex is involved. Older women are depicted as uniformly sexless or sexually unattractive. Most of this "humor" implies the impotence of older men and the ugliness of older women.

A mythology fed by misinformation surrounds late-life sexuality. The presumption is that sexual desire automatically ebbs with age—that it begins to decline when you are in your forties or even earlier, proceeds relentlessly downward (you are "losing it"), and eventually hits bottom (you are "over the hill") at some time between sixty and sixty-five. Thus an older woman who shows an evident, perhaps even a lusty, interest in sex is often assumed to be suffering from "emotional" problems; and if she is obviously in her right mind and sexually active, she runs the risk of being called "oversexed" or, more kindly, said to be clinging pathetically to her lost youth.

What is perceived as lustiness in young men is often seen as lechery in older men, a sign of inappropriate emotional lapse. Therefore, older men may find themselves the objects of sexual suspicion. Even simple affection can be misunderstood. An older man's show of warmth toward children other than his own grandchildren or those of his friends runs the risk of an assumption that it is sexually tinged. How real is this danger? According to crime statistics, child molesting, popularly associated with older men, is actually committed primarily by young men in their twenties.

From time to time everybody is caught up by accounts of older people who perform sexual feats "despite" their age. Newspapers relish them: 92-YEAR-OLD-MAN IS FATHER OF TWINS; WOMAN OF 73 AND MAN OF 76 ARRESTED BY POLICE IN LOVE NEST; JUDGE OF 81 MARRIES 22-YEAR-OLD SHOWGIRL; 72-YEAR-OLD WOMAN JAILED FOR ATTEMPTED PROSTITUTION. In the popular mind these older people walk the thin line between sexual heroics and indecency, with part of the public saying, "More power to them," and the remainder reacting with disgust. Everyone, however, reads the accounts with the mixture of revulsion and fascination reserved for the extraordinary and the bizarre.

Why are we still so negative about sex in later life and about older people in general? Much of this attitude is an outgrowth of our own fear of growing old and dying, and it has given rise to a prejudice we have called *ageism*, which is a systematic discrimination against people because they are old, just as racism and sexism discriminate for reasons of skin color and gender. The ageist sees older people in stereotypes: rigid, boringly talkative, senile, old-fashioned in morality and lacking in skills, useless, and with little redeeming social value. There's a fine irony in the fact that if the ageists live long enough they are going to end up being "old" themselves and the victims, in turn, of their own prejudice; their attitude will culminate in self-hatred. A great many older people have fallen into this trap, often at devastating cost to their personal happiness. And as far as sexuality is concerned, ageism says if you are getting old, you're finished.

Some of these attitudes are rooted in our relatively recent past. At the turn of the century, when the average life expectancy was forty-seven years, few older people lived to old age (about 3 percent) and fewer still were healthy enough to be sexually active. But today life expectancy is over seventy-six years and we have a large population of relatively healthy people over sixty-five. Of these, 95 percent live in the community, 80 percent or more can get around totally by themselves, and about 30 percent are still working part- or full-time. (We now term the age period sixty-five to seventy-four "early old age" and call that over seventy-five "later old age.") Indeed, centenarians are the fastest-growing age group. There are about seventy thousand today and conservative estimates are that there will be about 840,000 in 2050 and five million in 2100! Many of these oldest old are still surprisingly vigorous, as are a growing proportion of those who are somewhat younger. Yet we have not accepted these new realities, nor have popular attitudes caught up; the general image of late life still assumes frailty or decrepitude as par for the course.

If we combine these cultural attitudes with the

prevalent sexual criteria by which we are all measured, it is no wonder that older people may be confused and uncertain about sex! Both men and women worry about "wearing out" physically. They want to know what changes are to be expected with normal aging, whether there is reasonable hope for a physically healthy and active sex life, and whether lovemaking can be as good as it was when they were younger.

Men especially are victims of a lifelong excessive emphasis on physical performance. Masculinity is equated with physical prowess. Older men judge themselves and are judged by comparing the frequency and potency of their sexual performance with that of younger men. But these comparisons seldom place any value on experience and on the emotional quality of the sex. When measured by standards that are essentially athletic, older men are likely to be considered inferior. And so they often panic at the first sign of change: "Lately I've been troubled by the fact that I seem to take longer to have a good erection. Is something wrong? Am I becoming impotent? Will I be able to have a firm erection as I get older? Will sex be as pleasurable as when I was younger? Will my partner think I am inadequate?"

In terms of performance, women are under less pressure, of course, but they, too, worry about changes. They may report they are losing their "grip"—namely, the muscle strength in the vagina that enables them to hold a penis. The size of the vagina itself may change, and there may be problems with dryness as vaginal lubrication lessens. Some women begin to experience discomfort and/or pain during intercourse and want to know what to do to eliminate it. Both men and women without partners may worry about losing their sexual capacity altogether as a result of disuse.

The predominant pressure on women comes from what we term "sexual small-mindedness"—that widespread assumption that only the young are beautiful. Many older people believe this themselves. When a woman's hair turns gray and her skin changes and her body loses some of its earlier firmness and suppleness, she is very likely to see herself as unattractive. The idea of beauty desperately needs to be revised to include character, intelligence, expressiveness, knowledge, achievement, disposition, tone of voice and speech patterns, posture and bearing, warmth, personal style, social skills—all those personal traits that make each individual unique and that can be found at *any* age.

In late life we find just as many complaints between partners about sexual incompatibilities as at any other time: interest on one side and disinterest on the other, or passivity, or rebuffs, or failure to agree on the frequency of lovemaking. We get comments like the following all the time:

> I am in good health at age sixty-five and so is my sixty-three-year-old partner. She is a wonderful person, and she did a beautiful job rearing our five children. The problem—sex. On

my sixty-third birthday she did me the grand "favor" of sleeping with me. She then announced that from now on I'd better forget about sex because, as she put it, "We are too old to carry on like this." I don't feel old. I am still full of energy.

Problems also arise between couples when one partner is incapacitated or chronically ill and the other is healthy. If the healthy partner has active sexual needs, anger and irritation at being denied the opportunity to express sexuality often lead to guilt, as if one were lacking the appropriate concern and compassion for the ailing partner. The latter, in turn, may feel guilty at being unable to participate fully in lovemaking.

Tension in the later years often arises when those who are parents are inhibited by sons and daughters who find it uncomfortable to accept sexuality in their mothers and fathers. (We all agree that *our* parents were *never* interested in sex!) Many adult children continue to be bound by a primitive childhood need to deny their parents a sex life and to lock them into purely parental roles. For these individuals their parents never became fellow adults. Nor do negative emotions always derive from childhood. Adult avarice and selfishness, unhappily enough, are common. If one parent dies, children may deliberately try to prevent the surviving parent from meeting new friends and potential new partners in order to protect their inheritance. Any evidence of parental sexuality or romance threatens their hope for a financial legacy.

And what about the older lesbian, gay, bisexual, and transgender population (known collectively by the acronym LGBT), perhaps 5 to 10 percent of the population? We have included a section on such relationships and we join those who encourage dialogue and research on the specific concerns of this important older population. Older LGBT couples and individuals share many concerns and issues with older people generally, but they also deal with challenges specific to them.

We have now sketched out a number of ways—both positive and negative—in which individuals and society react to sexuality among older people. But what about those of you who are not particularly interested in sex? Numbers of older persons feel this way. We want to emphasize that sexual disinterest is a matter of concern *only* if you find it personally troubling or if it causes problems in relating to others. Some people were never significantly interested in sex even when younger, whether because of their biological makeup or, more often, as a result of social conditioning. For others sex represents emotional conflict resulting from or causing difficult relations with their partners. For them and their partners the opportunity to discontinue sex under the socially acceptable guise of "sexless old age" can be a great relief.

Others have simply grown tired of sex. From ancient Greece we hear a voice on this subject: "How well I remember the aged poet Sophocles' response to the question 'How does love sit with age, Sophocles: are you still the man you were?' 'Peace,' he replied. 'Most gladly have I escaped that of which you speak: I feel as if I had escaped from a mad and furious monster.' "*

If sex had been shared with the same partner routinely for years, many may now have compensated for its dullness by developing satisfying nonsexual activities. Other people may have stopped having sex because of disabilities or serious illnesses. When their health improved, there may have been no motivation to change what had become a comfortable habit. Sometimes an individual will have made a deliberate decision to share sex only with a particular partner, and thus, when illness or death intervenes, his or her experience of sex comes to a close. Other people view sex as solely procreative rather than as a pleasure, and feel their religion supports this conviction—so sexual expression ends with the completion of menopause. Self-imposed abstinence from sex may also be simply the continuation of a lifelong habit. This can often be traced back to frightening early experiences or to feelings that sex is forbidden and dangerous, and the avoidance of sex altogether may provide an adjustment that works reasonably well.

Whatever the reasons, it *is* possible to live a happy and satisfying life without sex if that is one's choice, and a good many older people do exactly that. The American

---

*From *Dialogues of Plato*, 4th ed. New York: Clarendon Press, 1953, p. 165.

emphasis on sexuality has had the effect of making many of the young and middle-aged feel guilty, inadequate, or incomplete if sex fails to play a central role in their lives; we do not want to place a similar burden on older people. Those who have neither a desire for nor an interest in sex, or who have deliberately chosen a lifestyle in which sexuality plays little or no part, are entitled to live the life they find most fulfilling.

On the other hand, those older people who do enjoy sex deserve encouragement and support, as well as necessary information, accurate diagnoses, and appropriate treatment if problems arise. Sexuality—the physical and emotional responsiveness to sexual stimuli—goes beyond the sexual urge and the sex act. For many older people it offers the opportunity to express not only passion but also affection, esteem, and loyalty. It provides affirmative evidence that one can count on one's body and its functioning. It allows people to assert themselves positively. It carries with it the possibility of excitement and romance; it expresses delight in being alive. It offers a continuous challenge to grow and change in new directions.

Chapter 2

✦

NORMAL PHYSICAL CHANGES IN SEXUALITY THAT OCCUR AS WE AGE

What happens to your body sexually as it ages? While there are significant changes in the physical and physiological aspects of sex as you age, such changes do not usually cause sexual problems unless disease, disability, or adverse drug effects interfere.

The act of sex is complex, encompassing the body, the mind, and the emotions. It involves the nervous and circulatory systems and the hormones as well as specific organs of the body. All of these participate in the sexual-response cycle, which includes sexual desire, followed by excitement or erotic arousal, orgasm or climax, and resolution or recovery. Both men and women experience similar sexual-response cycles.

People are stimulated sexually in a number of

ways—through sight, smell, sound, touch, thoughts, and feelings. The pelvic area reacts. Muscle tension, nerve activity, and congestion (filling of the blood vessels) occur, especially in the sexual or genital organs. The sex hormones that play an active role in this responsiveness are steroids, produced in the adrenal glands of both men and women and in the ovaries of women and the testes of men. Estrogen, one of the active female hormones, has a profound effect on the development and functioning of the female sex organs. Androgen (testosterone), the primary male hormone, appears to influence sexual desire in both men and women (women have small amounts of androgen) as well as sexual development and performance in men. It is the body's master gland, the pituitary, located in the brain, which affects the levels of all hormones, including the sex hormones. And as men and women age, the changes in these and other parts of their bodies affect their sexuality.

OLDER WOMEN

Most of the sexual changes in women can be directly traced to the decline of female hormones, especially estrogen, associated with menopause. Menopause, also called the "change of life" or "climacteric," is a physiological process that continues for several years and usually takes place anywhere between the ages of forty-five and fifty-five, with an average age of fifty to fifty-two. It involves decreases in estrogen levels from previously normal levels (prior to menopause) to about 20 percent of previous levels. Its most conspicuous sign is the cessation of menstruation. (Women who have had their ovaries surgically removed experience menopause abruptly.)

Although about 85 percent of women experience hot flashes and other menopausal symptoms during menopause, only about 20 to 30 percent actually seek medical attention for relief of such symptoms. It appears that many simply are not bothered enough by their symptoms to look for medical help; others are not aware of current medical interventions or cannot afford them. It is estimated that perhaps 25 percent of all women at the time of their menopause will have symptoms that, if left untreated, interfere in some significant way with their lives in middle age. Somewhat later, larger numbers of women will experience thinning of the vaginal walls as well as what is called "stress" or "urge" incontinence (see page 85). Much later, many but not most will develop the brittle bones and the tendency toward back pain and fractures that are typical of advanced osteoporosis, a condition exacerbated by the loss of estrogen in the postmenopausal years. Atherosclerosis in women in later life is also thought to be accelerated by the estrogen loss, although new controversy has recently surfaced on this subject. (Both osteoporosis and atherosclerosis in relation to estrogen will be discussed later in this chapter.) The following are examples of how differently menopause can affect individual women and their lifestyles.

Once her menopause began, Greta could hardly sleep at night. She would wake up drenched in sweat, totally alert, with her adrenaline flowing. It would be difficult to get back to sleep. When she did fall asleep again, she would awaken shortly thereafter in another devastating sweat that would leave her exhausted. After her sleep loss began to accumulate, she became irritable and depressed. She and her husband began to argue with each other. Greta grew more and more disconsolate and eventually went to her physician in despair, thinking she was losing her mind. Her internist tried tranquilizers. But eventually Greta saw her gynecologist, who prescribed short-term estrogen replacement therapy, which helped significantly. Her hot flashes, night sweats, irritability, and fatigue quickly disappeared. She and her gynecologist are now trying to decide whether long-term estrogen/progestin is indicated.

Florence, on the other hand, went through her menopause without apparent symptoms, as do about 15 percent of all women. In fact, the onset of menopause made her feel somewhat liberated. She and her husband had long since decided that three children were enough. Despite her use of contraception, she had always had a nagging concern that she might have an unwanted midlife pregnancy. Her husband, Philip, was delighted for her and for himself when they no longer had this concern and were free of the need to use birth control. Although Florence experienced a decrease in vaginal lubrication, as most women do after menopause, this was easily remedied with the use of vaginal lubricants.

Common symptoms resulting from the hormonal imbalance menopause causes may include hot flashes, headaches and neck aches, excessive fatigue, and feelings of emotional instability. Yet, none of these are inevitable, and when they do occur, they can often be greatly alleviated or sometimes relieved entirely through various medical and nonmedical treatments. Life stresses can also precipitate or exacerbate these menopausal symptoms, and under those circumstances psychological counseling can be helpful. But even when left untreated, certain menopausal symptoms, like hot flashes, usually subside spontaneously over time.

During or, more usually, following menopause, numbers of older women may begin to show signs of estrogen or sex-steroid changes that can affect their sexual functioning. Elizabeth, sixty-five, had experienced pain during intercourse in the first ten years after her menopause, which took place when she was fifty-one. She and her husband had given up making love once she turned sixty-one, much to her relief: The pain had not been worth the pleasure. When we saw her, we learned that her doctor had never inquired about any sexual problems, and that she in turn had been too embarrassed to discuss her vaginal pain and occasional vaginal bleeding. We quickly referred her for an evaluation and treatment. In her case, it simply meant using vaginal lubricants that could be purchased over the counter at her local pharmacy. Elizabeth and her husband began experimenting, tentatively at first, with resuming their sexual relationship. To her delight, Elizabeth discovered that she was pain-free.

Many women, like Elizabeth, do complain of a feeling of "dryness" or "loss of juices" in the vagina, particularly during sexual intercourse. (Vaginal lubrication produced by congestion of the blood vessels in the vaginal wall is the physiological equivalent of erection in the man.) Lubrication of the walls of the vagina begins to take longer as a woman grows older. This seems to be due both to the loss of the estrogen necessary to produce appropriate secretions and to changes in the structure of the vaginal wall itself, through which the secretions ooze. When this happens, intercourse may feel scratchy, rough, and eventually painful.

Typically, the lining of the vagina begins to thin and become easily irritated, leading to pain and sometimes to cracking and bleeding both during and after intercourse. The vagina is less able to absorb the shock of a thrusting penis. Such pain (dyspareunia) occurs especially if the intercourse is of a long duration, if lubrication is not adequate, or if intercourse follows a long period without sexual contact. Sometimes the shape of the vagina itself changes, becoming narrower, shorter, and less elastic, although generally it continues to be more than large enough for intercourse. Hormone replacement therapy has often been effective for protection against vaginal atrophy and dryness. (See pages 30–44 for a more detailed discussion of this therapy.) Vaginal lubricants are also extremely useful in decreasing or eliminating any pain.

Pain and discomfort of *any* kind in the vaginal area should always be taken seriously by women and their physicians since it obviously interferes with sexual pleasure and response. (It may also be a symptom of a more serious illness—in which case treatment of the underlying problem is indicated.) In many cases, but not always, physicians can tell during a vaginal exam whether a woman has vaginal atrophy severe enough to cause pain. Other causes of pain are vaginal dryness, endometriosis, a fixed retroverted uterus, a prolapsed ovary, or water in the fallopian tubes (hydrosalpinx)—all of which need attention.

With the loss of estrogen, the usually acidic vaginal secretions become less acidic, increasing the possibility of vaginal infection leading to burning, itching, and discharge. This condition is variously called estrogen-deficient, steroid-deficient, atrophic, or "senile" vaginitis. It *is* curable, and should be treated by a doctor. Home douching should not be attempted unless your doctor instructs you to do so for some specific medical purpose; it can confuse the diagnosis and may not, in any case, be an effective treatment.

Do not assume, however, that all vaginal itching and discharge reflect an estrogen deficiency. There should be a complete examination, including a Pap test, to rule out the possibility of a tumor of the reproductive tract. Allergies, contact dermatitis, and yeast and fungus infections (especially in diabetics) are other causes of itching; womb prolapse (fallen womb) may produce a vaginal discharge. A chronic condition known as vulvodynia (symptoms include pain, burning, inflammation, and/or rawness around the exterior of the genital area) is often misdiagnosed as a yeast infection, and requires a thorough evaluation and careful regimen of treatment. Antibiotics can suppress vaginal bacteria and allow yeast to overgrow, causing itching and discharge. Sexually transmitted diseases, such as trichomoniasis can cause itching, burning, and discharge.

First-time or recurrent vaginal infections should always be medically evaluated, since there are many types of candida with similar symptoms, in addition to other possible causes just described. Many women are able to use over-the-counter vaginal preparations (Gyne-Lotrimin, Monistat, and Femstat) if the condition has been diagnosed as the most common yeast infection, candida albicans. Other conditions require prescription medications. Home remedies such as eating yogurt or reducing sugar intake, although unreliable as a cure, may be of some help, especially in prevention, and certainly will cause no harm.

Preventive measures against vaginal infection include wearing cotton panties that "breathe," rather than nylon, spandex, or any tight-fitting undergarments that may tend to trap moisture, creating a medium for microorganisms to grow. When you use the toilet, wipe yourself from front to back to avoid contaminating the vaginal area with organisms from your bowel. Microbes that cause no trouble in the rectum can set off a painful inflammation once they enter the vagina. As previously mentioned, avoid douches, unless medically recommended. Make sure that you and your partner are clean before you have sex. Use lubricatory gels (water-based) for vaginal dryness. If you are taking antibiotics for any reason, have an over-the-counter vaginal ointment on hand in case vaginitis occurs.

Cystitis or inflammation of the bladder is another common problem. Bacterial or viral cystitis is often preventable. If you are subject to cystitis, carefully wash the vaginal area and your partner's penis with soap and water before sexual activity to reduce the possibility of infection. Drink water and urinate before lovemaking, since a full bladder is more easily irritated. Immediately after intercourse, drink large amounts of water and urinate frequently to flush out any disease agents. If you have a continued predisposition to such infection, your doctor may be able to prescribe preventive tablets (for example, sulfa, ampicillin, or nitrofurantoin) to take after sexual activity. If your symptoms persist, you may require a prolonged course of antibiotics. See your doctor.

Since the clitoral area of older women is often more sensitive to trauma or irritation, try to ensure that your sexual partner does not touch this area in a way that produces pain. Be frank in telling your partner what is pleasurable and what is not. Use a vaginal lubricant.

Some evidence suggests that diet is a factor in cystitis. Caffeine and alcohol may be irritants to the bladder. Diets high in refined sugars and starches (white flour, white rice, pasta, and the like) are possible factors in urinary tract problems, especially in diabetic women. Some believe that cranberry juice or vitamin C make urine more acidic and thus help prevent urinary tract infections.

Older women can develop what is sometimes called "honeymoon cystitis," an inflammation of the bladder resulting from bruising and jostling, or from exposure to semen and bacteria in the sensitive vaginal area after a period of sexual abstinence. With the thinning of the vaginal walls, the bladder and urethra (the tube through which the urine is passed) are less protected and may be irritated during intercourse. Again, drinking water and urinating prior to and after intercourse may be helpful. You may also alleviate the discomfort of honeymoon cystitis by changes in sexual positioning. The male should thrust his penis downward toward the back of the vagina and in the direction of the rectum, rather than toward the upper part of the vagina. This protects both the bladder and the delicate urethra.

Dorothy's inflammation of the bladder resulted from a weekend of sexual activity with her husband, which came after several years of abstinence. Her husband had had a heart attack two years before and had been fearful about engaging in sexual activity. Dorothy herself had been even more worried about the possible harmful effects. But their doctor had reassured them that they could safely resume sex. What he forgot to warn them of was the possibility of honeymoon cystitis, a kind of disuse problem. Fortunately, the situation quickly resolved itself; Dorothy's body soon adjusted to the presence of new bacterial substances resulting from intercourse.

Honeymoon cystitis is simply irritating at first, but when bacteria are present, it can become a full-fledged cystitis, characterized by an unrelenting, irresistible urge to urinate accompanied by a burning sensation. Advanced stages bring an increasingly painful burning during urination, waking at night to urinate, and, occasionally, blood in the urine. Such infections require prompt medical attention.

Women's physical capacity for sexual arousal often continues throughout life, assuming the absence of illness or other factors that typically interfere. As women age they might notice that the clitoris becomes slightly reduced in size, although this is not always the case. The lips of the vagina (the labia) may become less firm. The covering of the clitoris and the fat pad in the hair-covered pubic area lose some of their fatty tissue, leaving the clitoris less protected and more easily irritated. However, clitoral stimulation continues to be a source of sexual sensation and orgasm.

Women in good health who were able to have orgasms in their younger years can often continue doing so until very late in life—well into their eighties or even later. Indeed, some women begin to have orgasms for the first time as they grow older. The lack of orgasmic ability earlier in life does not necessarily mean that such a pattern will continue if a woman eventually learns how to understand and manage her own sexual response. What is unclear, however, is whether the length of time required to reach orgasm changes as women age. Nor do we know for certain whether age is associated with duration and intensity of an orgasm. For some, shorter-lasting orgasms and spasms in the uterus, when they occur, may be evidence of a hormonal imbalance or other factors. Finally, little is known definitively about sexual desire as women grow older.

A condition called "female sexual dysfunction" (FSD) has begun appearing regularly in the psychiatric and self-help literature. The *1994 Diagnostic and Statistical Manual of Mental Disorders*, 4th edition (DSM IV), defines four categories of FSD: 1) desire disorders; 2) female sexual arousal disorder; 3) female orgasmic disorder; and 4) female sexual pain disorders. In an article published in 1999 in *The Journal of the American*

Medical Association, nearly half of American women of all ages were described as suffering from FSD (compared to 31 percent of men with erectile dysfunction). Questions abound as to the validity of the FSD diagnosis, just as earlier labels of "frigidity" and other terms failed to inspire confidence as adequate descriptions of problematic female sexual functioning. The DSM IV classification scheme does not note physical organic causes of FSD, nor does it recognize social or societal issues. Further, the sizable numbers of women described as suffering from the FSD syndrome are suspect, particularly in view of current pharmaceutical company interest in opening up a vast new female market for drug therapy. Considerable research is needed to separate out general sexual problems for women from a host of factors that now appear to be subsumed under the diagnosis of FSD.

To summarize, except for the effects of estrogen loss after menopause, the normal physical changes that accompany aging appear to interfere very little with a female's sexual ability. Reports of a decline in women's sexual interest as a consequence of aging per se are controversial. What is clear is that diseases, physical disabilities, medications, surgery, excessive alcohol, or tobacco can be culprits in lessened sexual desire and sexual response. There are also psychological factors that lead to defensive or protective sexual behaviors. For example, the frequency of sexual activity for a woman is often affected by her partner's age, health, and level of sexual interest and functioning, rather than a reflection of her own reduced interest or capacity. (Remember that most married women outlive their husbands. Therefore, husbands usually grow frail before their partners do.)

We want to emphasize that many older women show a spirited and continuing interest in love and sexuality. Here is a letter we received from a seventy-two-year-old:

It's about time that someone acknowledged and brought out of the closet the subject of sexual desire and activity for those of us in our later years. I live in a senior citizens' apartment building where 95 percent of the tenants are women. There are four or five widowers here, but none of them is currently being pursued by a woman. Isn't this pathetic? People here are too sedentary. Unfortunately, none of these men is personally appealing to me or I would take action. . . . At my age I still consider myself attractive enough for any man, maybe even one a few years younger than myself. All I need to know now is "where the boys are."

Our reply:

Thank you for your wonderful letter. It is great to hear from readers as lively and enthusiastic as you. We share your concerns about "where the boys are." As you know, there is no easy answer to this question. Men will sooner or later have to learn to live healthier lives so they don't die off so quickly! In the meantime, it is a delight to hear from someone as spirited as you, even when an interesting man is not available.

TREATMENT OF POSTMENOPAUSAL CHANGES

REGULAR SEXUAL ACTIVITY

Although still subject to debate, there is some evidence that regular sexual activity helps preserve functioning, especially vaginal lubricatory ability, and may even stimulate estrogen production. Sexually active women also seem to have less vaginal atrophy. The regular muscle contractions during sexual activity and orgasm do maintain vaginal muscle tone, and it is thought that intercourse helps preserve the shape and size of the vaginal space.

Yet, following the death or illness of a partner,

many women find themselves without the opportunity for sexual contact. If it is personally acceptable, self-stimulation (masturbation) can be effective in preserving lubricating ability and the muscle tone that maintains the size and shape of the vagina. In addition, it can release tension, stimulate sexual appetite, and contribute to general well-being. Self-stimulation is probably more common among younger women because they have grown up in a less restrictive sexual atmosphere. But it seems clear that it is being practiced by women of all ages with growing frequency, lessened anxiety, and considerable physical benefit. In fact, masturbation is increasingly viewed not only as a response to the loss of sexual contact with a partner but also as a natural and ongoing supplementary activity within a relationship.

HORMONE REPLACEMENT THERAPY

The popularity of estrogen replacement therapy (ERT) and the estrogen/progestin combination known as hormone replacement therapy (HRT) has had its ups and downs in recent years. Estrogen was first used to treat the problems of menopause in the late 1940s. The use of estrogen in its most popular form, Premarin, gained momentum throughout the 1960s and the mid-1970s, fueled by physician Robert Wilson's popular book,

Feminine Forever. ERT was promoted as a protection against hot flashes, backache, memory loss, vaginal atrophy, depression, lowered sex drive, and such general aging signs as wrinkles and gray hair. Common side effects were thought to be occasional dose-related uterine bleeding and minor complaints of nausea, fluid retention, weight gain, and increased susceptibility to vaginal yeast infection. By 1975, about six million women were receiving ERT.

ERT usage declined sharply after five studies in 1975–1976 showed it was associated with an increased risk of endometrial cancer (cancer affecting the lining of the uterus)—especially if ERT had been given for more than five years. Both women and their physicians became wary. But after several more years, researchers learned that adding progestin (a synthetic form of the female hormone progesterone) counters, and perhaps avoids altogether, the buildup in the endometrium that leads to endometrial cancer. With this news, the use of HRT, this time combining estrogen—in lower doses than formerly—and progestin, began to climb again. By the year 2000, approximately forty million women had reached menopause, and more than seventeen million were receiving some form of HRT (ten million on estrogen alone and seven million on some combination of hormones, including estrogen).

Newer developments have brought added promise, as well as controversy and challenge, to the question of hormone use. Until recently, studies—including the ongoing Boston-based Nurses' Health Study of 48,470 postmenopausal women with no previous heart disease—supported earlier observations that estrogen has preventive and life-lengthening effects against a number of the major disease killers and disablers of older women. This catapulted ERT into use as a treatment for conditions other than menopause. Growing numbers of women over fifty began reassessing estrogen use as a possible lifelong protection against heart disease, the greatest cause of death among women, and osteoporosis, one of the major causes of female disability in later life. Suggestions that estrogen might also be protective against Alzheimer's disease added to the enthusiasm for hormone replacement. Estrogen in the form of Premarin became the best-selling prescription drug in America.

However, a possible link between estrogen and the development of breast cancer and perhaps ovarian cancer continues to be enormously worrisome to many women. Further, we currently know little about the long-term effects of adding progestin to the hormone replacement regimen, including whether it interferes with any protections that estrogen may prove to have against the diseases of later life.

The biology of menopause, which is still not clearly understood, and these unresolved questions regarding postmenopausal HRT are now receiving increased attention at the National Institutes of Health (specifically the recently concluded Postmenopausal

Estrogen/Progestin Interventions Trial, or PEPI study, at the National Heart, Lung, and Blood Institute, as well as the ongoing, nationwide Women's Health Initiative) and elsewhere. The goal is to produce substantially more reliable information on hormone replacement for women and their physicians. Women and their health-care providers are eagerly awaiting answers from the Women's Health Initiative's clinical trials involving more than twenty-seven thousand women age fifty and older. Results should become available in 2005. (Using Google as a search engine on the Internet, simply type in *Women's Health Initiative* to immediately access the Web site.)

The growing longevity of American women makes it imperative that the issues surrounding HRT use are clarified. Altogether, with the aging of the baby-boom generation of women, nearly seventy million American women are now postmenopausal.

A Menopause Guidebook, published by the North American Menopause Society (NAMS), P.O. Box 94527, Cleveland, OH 44101, phone: 440-442-7559, is available free on the NAMS Web site or by writing or calling NAMS.

For a positive position on estrogen use, see *Estrogen: A Complete Guide to Menopause and Hormone Replacement Therapy* by Lila E. Nachtigall, M.D., and Joan R. Heilman, New York: HarperResource, 2000. For an opposing view, especially with regard to heart disease, see "Hormones and Heart Disease: Medical Bias

Disregards Best Evidence," *National Women's Health Network* (September/October 2000).

Benefits of Estrogen (with Provisos)

The known risks and benefits of HRT must be evaluated individually by each woman and her physician (easy to say but frustrating for many, in view of currently conflicting and inadequate information on HRT effects). HRT provides short-term benefits for many women with troublesome symptoms directly related to menopause. It appears that there also may be broader long-term health benefits from estrogen use, although it depends on the disease states under consideration, and further study is clearly warranted. Risks, especially in connection with possible involvement with breast and ovarian cancer, have created anxiety. (The latest evidence suggests that long-term estrogen use—five to ten years or more—may increase the risk of cancer, although there is still no consensus on the subject. To further complicate the picture, several recent studies found the risk higher when estrogen and progestin were used together, rather than estrogen alone.) Physicians are markedly confused and divided on the subject. We will attempt to give an overall view of what is currently known.

Protection against Menopausal Symptoms

Estrogen replacement is very effective in alleviating and, in most cases, eliminating many of the more immediate symptoms of menopause, especially hot flashes ("night sweats"), vaginal dryness, and thinning of the vaginal walls with accompanying pain, discomfort, and even bleeding during sexual intercourse. And when hot flashes disappear, insomnia, irritability, and depression resulting from lack of sleep often improve dramatically. Some women also report fewer headaches and memory problems than they had during the menopausal period.

Protection against Heart Disease

A number of studies have found that oral estrogen increases high-density lipoproteins (HDLs—the "good" cholesterol) while decreasing the low-density lipoproteins (LDLs—the dangerous cholesterol). When administered in the form of a "patch," cream, or gel, estrogen still lowers LDLs, but has little or no effect on HDLs. These effects on cholesterol and other effects on blood vessels are thought to prevent the formation of fatty deposits in the arteries that interfere with blood flow and can lead to both heart attacks and strokes. Other studies have shown additional benefits for the heart. This has been welcome news, since heart disease is the leading cause of death in postmenopausal women beginning around age sixty.

However, more recently, preliminary results from the large HRT trial of the Women's Health Initiative suggest that estrogen use may result in a slightly higher risk of heart attacks and strokes in the first two years of use, with the effect diminishing as use continues. These results are not definitive, and it won't be known if they hold up when final study findings are released somewhere around 2005. Other recent research indicates that *women with already-existing heart disease* showed no benefit from estrogen use. There has been little investigation of whether estrogen may be helpful in preventing heart disease from developing in the first place, although a number of researchers are less hopeful than in the past.

Reports that women taking estrogen live longer than those that do not have also come under scrutiny. Critics point out that women taking estrogen are also less likely to smoke and more likely to exercise and eat healthy diets than women who are not on estrogen. Thus, their longevity may be related to better health habits rather than estrogen.

Protection against Osteoporosis

Osteoporosis is a demineralizing disease that leads to bone loss and fractures. It affects six times as many older women as older men, and 40 percent of all older women show symptoms of the disease. It is the cause of bone fractures in 40 percent of women over seventy and can lead to broken hips, permanent disability, and death. Estrogen has the reputation of slowing the rapid bone loss that occurs during menopause and helps to prevent the thinning of the bones that leads to osteoporosis. However, recent studies are beginning to question these contentions, with recommendations shifting to the use of non-hormonal drugs such as alendronate sodium (Fosamax) for protection against osteoporosis.

Protection against Alzheimer's Disease

Early epidemiological research suggested that estrogen might improve the memory of women with Alzheimer's disease. Unfortunately, a recent large and long-term study reported in *The Journal of the American Medical Association* (February 23, 2000) has failed to support this hope for women with already well-established Alzheimer's. Nonetheless scientists emphasize that estrogen may still prove useful in preventing the disease or delaying its onset. Researchers at the National Institute on Aging, using neuroimaging technology, report that postmenopausal women taking estrogen "age differently and have significantly greater blood flow to areas involved in memory formation than the brains of women who do not receive hormone replacement" (National Institute on Aging news release, June 27, 2000). Further clinical trials are currently underway.

Benefits of Progesterone (Progestin) Therapy—Without Estrogen

Progesterone or synthetic progestin is given alone to women with menopausal symptoms who cannot or do not wish to take estrogen. It is especially used to counter hot flashes, although it cannot compare to estrogen in effectiveness. The dosage is usually 2.5 milligrams of oral medroxyprogesterone (Provera) per day. The Food and Drug Administration (FDA) has approved a version called Megace (megestrol acetate) for women who have had breast cancer. Depo-Provera is another form of the drug, and must be injected every three months. Progesterone is also available as a moisturizing cream and as a capsule designed to melt under the tongue.

Risks and Problems Associated with HRT

Estrogen Risks

There is evidence that estrogen replacement can accelerate the development of preexisting estrogen-dependent cancers and of noncancerous fibroid tumors in the uterus. There is currently no clear evidence, however, that estrogen encourages the growth of new cancers, especially when a woman has been using estrogen for less than five years. Estrogen may also increase the risk of gallbladder disease, blood clots, hypertension, and PMS-like symptoms.

Controversy over estrogen and ovarian cancer surfaced in March 2001, with a study suggesting that ovarian cancer rates doubled with estrogen use. However, women were reminded that the chances of dying of ovarian cancer are extremely low (1.7 percent over a woman's lifetime), so that twice the risk is still very low. No increased risk was found among those using estrogen for periods under ten years. Progestin use does not appear to have been studied in this research.

Who should *not* use estrogen? If you have any of the following conditions, your doctor will probably advise you to avoid taking estrogen:

- A known or suspected breast or uterine cancer or any other tumor that is stimulated by estrogen. Some physicians take the position that fibrocystic breast changes, fibroid tumors of the uterus, and endometriosis are also contraindications to taking estrogen.
- A strong family history of estrogen-dependent cancers.
- Diabetes, although this is a "relative" contraindication, since there is evidence that estrogen does not worsen, and may even improve, control of blood sugar.
- Blood clots of any kind, including thrombophlebitis, embolism, stroke, or heart attack.
- Chronic or acute liver disease.
- Abnormal or unexplained genital bleeding.
- Allergic reaction to estrogen.

Your doctor should also be cautious if you have high levels of fat (triglycerides) in the blood, severe varicose veins, or very high blood pressure. (Note: Estrogen raises triglycerides but lowers cholesterol.)

Progestin Problems

When progestin is added to the hormone replacement regimen as a protection against uterine cancer, some women experience side effects such as weight gain, abdominal bleeding, headaches, irritability, and breast tenderness. Bleeding is usually eliminated after the first few months when progestin is given on a continuous, low-dosage basis. As described earlier, there is also evidence that progestin, especially when given in larger doses, may interfere with any protective effect, if any, that estrogen provides against heart disease. Some believe that what is called "micronized natural progesterone" (sold under the name Prometrium), made from soy or wild yam, is superior to synthetic progestins and helps avoid deleterious side effects, although definitive research is lacking.

Remember that not all women on HRT take progestin. For example, those who have had hysterectomies do not need progestin, since they have no uteruses. Other women, for a variety of reasons, choose to use estrogen alone, without progestin. It is strongly urged that such women have semiannual or at least yearly endometrial biopsies (a simple procedure that can be done in your doctor's office). Such biopsies can detect endometrial cancer in its early stages, when it is curable through hysterectomy.

How HRT Is Administered

Research is beginning to suggest that women's need for estrogen may shift with age, with more needed during the menopausal period and less later. Lower dose regimens may be the wave of the future—an advantage in terms of overall side effects and concerns about breast cancer (and possibly, the newest findings on heart disease), but a possible disadvantage for certain other long-term benefits. However, low-dose therapy has been encouraging in terms of control of hot flashes and other symptoms. Current studies are using half of usual amounts of estrogen and progestin and some think the dosages will go even lower into "ultralow" categories. This will be a particular advantage to older women who begin to take HRT later in life in their seventies and eighties and who may find higher doses problematic. Another advantage is that estrogen doses may drop so low that the threat of endometrial cancer is removed and progestin is no longer needed. Studies in this area are ongoing and promising for safer HRT use.

Currently, estrogen may be taken in several different ways: orally in pills, by means of a transdermal skin patch, in a vaginal cream, or by injection (rare). When a woman still has her uterus, progestin is typically added, taken orally in pill form. (Note: Many women are not aware that progestin is best taken at bedtime because it can cause feelings of general fatigue.)

In the past, *Estrogen pills*, in combination with *progestin*, have often been given in cyclic manner: one estrogen pill (0.625 milligrams each) a day for twenty-five days each month, with progestin pills (5 to 10 milligrams each) added for the last ten to fourteen days of this period, followed by five to seven days with no pills.

In order to avoid the bleeding associated with HRT, a more popular option is "combined-continuous" hormone therapy, involving an estrogen pill and a low-dosage progestin pill (for example, 2.5 milligrams) each day, without any breaks.

Various other combinations of estrogen and progestin are also used, including drug holidays in which one or both drugs are temporarily stopped. One schedule is to take progestin for ten days at a time only once every three to four months. Others believe that taking progestin as little as twice a year is enough to prevent endometrial cancer.

The *transdermal skin patch* looks like a Band-Aid and is applied to the skin of the abdomen, hip, or upper thigh. It delivers estrogen directly into the bloodstream through the skin, and is changed twice a week. The patch is used for twenty-five days each month. Unlike the pill, this form of estrogen bypasses the liver and the digestive system and therefore does not have beneficial effects on HDL (good) cholesterol levels. It still lowers LDL (bad) cholesterol quite effectively. Estrogen in this form is especially useful for women with liver problems that would be complicated by estrogen.

Vaginal estrogen cream is applied directly to the vagina to help counteract the dryness and loss of elasticity that many women experience during and after menopause. Its main purpose is to make sexual intercourse more comfortable. Although the estrogen in the cream is absorbed into the rest of the body through the bloodstream, the amount is thought to be small. However, it may offer protection against urinary tract infections.

If you are using estrogen cream to counteract vaginal dryness and restore lubrication, apply it at least one hour before sexual intercourse. In this way, you will have given your body a chance to absorb the hormone and thus lessen the possibility that your partner will be exposed to it during intercourse. Estrogen can cause increases in breast size and other undesirable effects in men.

The *vaginal ring (Estring)* is an estradiol-releasing vaginal ring designed for treating postmenopausal atrophy of the vagina (causing dryness, burning, itching, and difficult or painful intercourse) and/or lower urinary tract (difficulty urinating or urinary urgency). A new ring is inserted every three months.

Vagifem is a vaginal estrogen tablet for relief of vaginal dryness or pain associated with menopause. One tablet is inserted into the vagina daily for the first two weeks, then twice a week after that.

Selective estrogen receptor modulators (SERMs), also known as "designer estrogens," are being developed to bypass or lessen some of the negative effects of estrogen. Raloxifene (Evista), tamoxifen (Nolvadex), and idoxifene are some of the most commonly used SERMs. However, they do not prevent hot flashes, nor do they have several of the other beneficial effects of estrogen. Tamoxifen also increases the risk of uterine cancer. On the other hand, these SERMs may be especially valuable for women at high risk for breast cancer, since they do not stimulate breast tissue.

Testosterone Therapy

While estrogen can be beneficial in a number of ways after menopause, it does not have a direct effect upon sexual desire. If loss of libido is a prime complaint for a woman, small amounts of testosterone may improve her sexual appetite. Natural testosterone levels may decline in some women after menopause. "Low levels" of testosterone have been described as less than 30 milligrams per 100 milliliters of blood plasma, measurable through a simple blood test. However, experts caution that measurements may be meaningless at such low levels and the best test is often to try the hormone to observe its effects.

Testosterone use is still somewhat controversial, largely because of concerns about untoward side effects. Nevertheless, physicians and researchers tend to agree that tiny amounts (1 to 2 milligrams per dose once a day) may bring about increased sexual desire while avoiding cholesterol or heart attack risk as well as the masculinizing effects of facial hair growth, acne, and voice deepening. Physicians may also prescribe testosterone along with HRT (Estratest tablets combine 1.25 milligrams of testosterone with 0.625 milligrams of estrogen) to help control unusually persistent hot flashes (FDA approved for this use) as well as the breast tenderness and headaches experienced by some women taking estrogen.

Testosterone therapy is particularly important to consider for women who have had their ovaries removed before menopause or who have experienced an early menopause. As just described, considerable research also indicates that women in the immediate postmenopause period may benefit from its use. Less is known about the effects of testosterone on much older women, although reported increases in bone mass while using it may help protect against osteoporosis.

Viagra—Does It Work for Women?

The Pfizer drug company's first controlled study of nearly six hundred European, American, and Canadian women, presented in May 2000, found that Viagra performed no better than a placebo. Prior to using Viagra, the women research subjects' primary complaints included low levels of desire and arousal, inability to achieve orgasm, and painful dryness during intercourse. Although Viagra increased blood flow to the genitals, it did little else to improve sexual response. Researchers concluded, "sexual dysfunctions in women are more complex" than those found in men, principally because "when women talk about problems with arousal they are often talking about different things," from genital arousal to "mental excitement." One can ascertain from this that men primarily emphasize erectile capacity ("is my penis working?") while women bring together a wider, intertwined range of concerns that involve physical ability for arousal and orgasm, relationships with partners, and personal psychology—all of which form the "mental set" necessary for female sexual response.

A related outcome of the Pfizer clinical trials of women was a recognition that there is as yet no reliable way to accurately measure female sexual response. In contrast to the relatively simple manner in which male erectile capacity can be tracked, female sexuality requires a more complex set of measurements. Current attempts by Pfizer include a newly developed, self-administered questionnaire called the Index of Female Sexual Function (patterned after the International Index of Erectile Function designed for men), as well as an experimental use of the magnetic resonance imaging scan (MRI) combined with an injection of a contrast fluid to measure blood flow to the genitals, while watching an erotic video. Pfizer acknowledges that neither approach represents a validated, widely accepted assessment tool for measuring female sexual function.

In spite of negative research results, anecdotal reports of Viagra use for women have been somewhat more positive. A few researchers are experimenting with off-label use of the drug and an unknown number of women are trying it on their own, with or without prescriptions from their doctors. Irwin Goldstein, urologist at the Boston University School of Medicine, has stated the belief that Viagra may eventually prove beneficial to two groups of women: those who are experiencing a lack of sexual desire as a side effect of antidepressants and postmenopausal women who report dryness, painful intercourse, and diminished ability to reach orgasm. Others disagree, doubtful that Viagra can improve orgasmic capacity simply by increasing blood flow to the genitals.

Another effect of Viagra has been the burst of new attention to female sexuality, especially by drug companies searching for sexually oriented drugs with the hope of marketing them to a huge and previously untapped group of customers. A host of drugs are already in various stages of testing. As an example, two companies, Vivus and Wysor, have received similar patents for prostaglandin-based gels designed to increase blood flow to the female genitals.

The first medical device (called Eros CTD) designed to help women with "sexual dysfunction" was approved by the Food and Drug Administration in May 2000. It works on a principle similar to the vacuum pumps used by men to achieve erection.

ALTERNATIVE MENOPAUSAL TREATMENTS

Because of risk factors or negative physical reactions, not all women can use HRT. Others are strongly opposed to hormone use for reasons that range from the personal to the philosophical, including a conviction that the menopause is a natural phenomenon and should not be considered a medical issue.

The U.S. Congressional Office of Technology Assessment (no longer in existence) officially approved only one nonhormonal drug for the treatment of such menopausal symptoms as hot flashes. This is Bellergal-S, which contains the sedative phenobarbital and belladonna. Yet according to studies, Bellergal helps only about half of the women who take it and is potentially addictive. Further, it may cause digestive problems and blurred vision. Today it is seldom used.

"Natural" remedies such as vitamins and herbs, as well as certain diets, exercise, and biofeedback have not been well studied, but anecdotal reports and a few clinical investigations indicate that some of them may be helpful for some women. Vitamin E in daily doses of 400 to 800 International Units is one of the most popular alternative menopausal remedies. (Higher doses may be harmful.) Many women who have tried it believe it to be useful in reducing the frequency and severity of hot flashes. Vitamin B_6 in daily doses of 50 to 200 milligrams may help with various menopausal symptoms experienced by some women, such as emotional instability, tiredness, loss of libido, depression, and loss of mental concentration. However, more than 200 milligrams daily may cause neurological problems.

Black cohosh, an American Indian remedy, may have an effect on hot flashes, although side effects may include upset stomach, headaches, dizziness, and weight gain. It may lower blood pressure. Dong quai, a highly popular Chinese herb, has not been found to be effective in reducing hot flashes and may have dangerous side effects. (In China it is apparently used in combination with other herbs, not by itself.)

Ginseng contains compounds that mimic estrogen, and is available in capsules, root form, or as a tea, powder, or syrup. Its effectiveness has not been reliably tested, but it has had a reputation as a menopausal remedy for a long time. It can be dangerous for diabetics who are on medications because it may lower blood sugar. It may also build up the lining of the uterus, much like estrogen (without progestin) does.

Foods such as alfalfa, flaxseed, cherries, sesame seeds, and many others contain plant estrogens or phytoestrogens. Because of the weak amounts of estrogen they contain, there is little evidence that phytoestrogens are effective in combating menopausal symptoms. Soy may be modestly helpful in lowering cholesterol after menopause, but studies have not demonstrated that it is useful in reducing hot flashes or bone loss. There is also a question as to whether soy (as well as black cohosh mentioned earlier) and other foods with phytoestrogens stimulate some breast tumors or endometrial cancers. When soy is used, experts recommend that it is eaten in the form of natural foods, rather than taken as a soy supplement which may far exceed normal dietary amounts of phytoestrogens. Saint-John's wort, kava, wild yam, red clover, and valerian are other preparations that in low doses may be fairly safe, but their effectiveness is unknown and side effects can be troublesome.

It should be noted that many women are self-medicating with alternative medicines in amounts that far exceed those found in natural foods or in traditional medicine practices. Nothing is known about the effects of such giant dosages. Others are taking combinations of supplements and herbs that have never been tried before and whose chemical interactions are unknown. Scientists like Dr. Fredi Kronenberg, director of the Center for Complementary and Alternative Medicine at the Columbia University College of Physicians and Surgeons in New York City, warn that such experimentation is dangerous.

Biofeedback techniques for regulating body temperature may hold promise for controlling hot flashes, but such techniques have yet to be developed for this purpose. Acupuncture and relaxation therapies are also being studied as menopausal treatments.

Lastly, various drugs such as clonidine have been shown in studies to reduce the severity and frequency of hot flashes in some patients. But unpleasant side effects may occur with their use (e.g. rare lowering of normal blood pressure) and other menopausal symptoms such as vaginal dryness and bone loss are not relieved. Anti-depressants such as Prozac, Paxil, and Effexor have also been found to reduce hot flashes. This may be particularly useful for women with prior breast cancer or for those who cannot otherwise take estrogen. Further studies are underway.

PREVENTION PRACTICES

All menopausal women, regardless of whether they use HRT, can improve their health and lower the risk of heart disease, osteoporosis, and other health problems by the following measures. Impressive evidence is accumulating that good health habits are the critical underlying factor in avoiding disease and disability and as an adjunct in treating already existing conditions. Many consider them to be the *first line of defense*, before anything else. The health habits include:

- A diet low in saturated fat, with adequate calcium and fiber (see Chapter 7).
- Regular exercise (see Chapter 7).
- Moderate alcohol use and no smoking.
- Stress-reduction measures.
- Regular medical tests, including Pap tests and mammograms. Both tests should be done

annually throughout life after the age of fifty, for the early detection of cancer. (Medicare now provides reimbursement for Pap tests and mammograms.)
- Monthly breast self-exams.

OVER-THE-COUNTER REMEDIES FOR VAGINAL DISCOMFORT

If you are experiencing vaginal dryness or discomfort, whether or not you are using HRT, a simple lubricant that dissolves in water (K-Y Jelly, Astroglide, Slip, HR Lubricating Jelly, or Ortho Personal Lubricants, for example) can be placed in the vagina immediately before intercourse. A moisturizing gel in tampon form called Replens, available over the counter, can be inserted vaginally three times a week to build up a continuously moist layer in the vagina. The advantage of moisturizers (like Replens, Lubrin, and Gyne-Moistrin) versus lubricants is that they can be inserted in advance and therefore do not interfere with sexual spontaneity. Do *not* use oil-based lubricants such as petroleum jelly, mineral oil, baby oil, or body lotion because they do not dissolve in water and can be a vehicle for vaginal infection. (They can also break down the latex in condoms in seconds, creating tears and breaks.) Remember also that there can be factors other than menopause that lead to vaginal dryness. These include use of antidepressants, antihistamines and certain decongestants, and other medications that can dry out the mucus membranes of the vagina. Condoms, even the prelubricated ones, may cause problems unless additional lubricants are used. Emotional and physical stress can also be a factor. It is estimated that up to one-third of all women regularly use a lubricant during sexual intercourse.

OLDER MEN

Most men secretly begin to worry about sexual aging at some time in their thirties, when they start to compare their present level of sexual activity with their previous performance as teenagers and very young adults. These worries tend to accelerate in the forties and fifties and reach a peak in the sixties as they continue to observe definite sexual changes.

What changes do men notice? Quite simply, their sexual organs don't respond quite as quickly as they did at a younger age. Fred, a man in his late fifties, noticed these changes but didn't realize that they were normal and, most importantly, manageable. Instead, he panicked: "I'm definitely slower about having an erection—and quite frankly, this is unnerving. I have been divorced for several years, and recently on a business trip I stopped to see a woman with whom I had had a wonderful affair some twenty years ago. We found we were still attracted to each other. But when we attempted to make love, it took me forever to get things underway. She took this as a sign that I wasn't interested in her, and we ended up not having sex at all. I was totally humiliated and so was she. What a disaster!"

Lacking a full understanding of normal sexual changes with age, men misinterpret them as alarming and as either the onset of impotence or its future inevitability. "From a psychosexual point of view," say Masters and Johnson, "the male over age fifty has to contend with one of the great fallacies of our culture. Every man in this age group is arbitrarily identified by both public and professional alike as sexually impaired."

Aging alone does not cause sexual impairment. Potency is the man's sexual capacity for intercourse. Impotence, now more properly called erectile dysfunction, is the temporary or permanent incapacity to have an erection sufficient to carry out the sexual act. (Do not confuse sterility with erectile dysfunction. Sterility means infertility or the incapacity to father children.) What is normal erectile functioning for one man may not be normal for another. There are variations in the frequency of erection and the length of time a man maintains an erection. Such individual differences often continue over many years, defining unique personal patterns. Therefore, comparisons of a man's present sexual status must be made in terms of *his* past history and not in terms of some generalized "standard" involving comparisons with other men. Most sex therapists do not consider impotence or erectile dysfunction to be a problem unless it occurs in at least 25 percent or more of sexual encounters with the same partner.

While individual variation from man to man must be taken into account, there are a number of gradual and fairly predictable processes that affect sexuality and are associated with chronological aging. An older man ordinarily takes longer to obtain an erection than a younger man. The difference is a matter of minutes after sexual stimulation rather than a few seconds. The erection may also not be quite as large, straight, and hard as in previous years. Once the man is fully excited, however, his erection will usually be sturdy and reliable, particularly if this was the pattern in earlier life. *The critical point to remember is that increased manual stimulation of the penis by the man himself or his partner is often all that is necessary to promote and maintain arousal.* Visual stimulation may also be helpful—such as videos and films now widely available in neighborhood video stores, hotel rooms, and elsewhere.

The lubrication that appears prior to ejaculation (Cowper's gland secretory activity) decreases or disappears completely as men age, but this has little effect on sexual performance. There is also a reduction in the volume of seminal fluid, and this results in a decrease in the need to ejaculate. Younger men produce 3 to 5 milliliters of semen (about one teaspoon) every twenty-four hours, while men past fifty produce 2 to 3 milliliters. This can be a decided advantage in lovemaking, since lessened ejaculatory pressure means that the older man can delay ejaculation more easily and thus make love longer. This in turn extends his own enjoyment and enhances the possibility of orgasm/pleasure for his partner.

The experience of orgasm may begin to feel somewhat different with age. The younger man is aware of a few pleasurable seconds, just before ejaculation, when he can no longer control himself. As ejaculation occurs, powerful contractions are felt and the semen spurts with a force that can carry it one to two feet from the tip of the penis. With an older man there may be a briefer period of awareness before ejaculation or no such period at all. (In some men, however, this period actually lengthens because of spasms in the prostate.) The orgasm itself is generally less explosive, in that the semen is propelled a shorter distance and the contractions are less forceful. *None* of these physiological changes interferes with the aging man's experiencing totally satisfying orgasmic pleasure, even when the preejaculation stage is altered or completely missing.

The forcefulness of orgasm also lessens naturally when a couple voluntarily prolongs their lovemaking before orgasm. Many older men become aware that they have a choice of an extended period of sexual pleasure with a milder orgasm or a briefer session with a more intense orgasm.

Whereas younger men can usually have another

ejaculation in a matter of minutes after orgasm, the older man generally must wait a longer period of time (the refractory period), from several hours up to several days, before an ejaculation is again possible. In addition, the older man may rapidly lose his erection following orgasm, sometimes so quickly that the penis literally slips out of the vagina. This is not a sign of impairment of the penis and its erectile capacity, but simply a physical change that requires a mental adjustment.

Older men should not fall into the common trap of measuring manhood by the frequency with which they can carry intercourse through to ejaculation. Some men over sixty are physically satisfied with one or two ejaculations per week because of the decrease of semen production, while others are more active. Still others, particularly if they were less sexually active earlier in life, do not ejaculate frequently or even regularly. Each man should find a level of ejaculatory frequency he is comfortable with. Remember also that lovemaking need not be limited to ejaculatory ability. Men who are knowledgeable and comfortable about themselves may have intercourse as frequently as they wish but ejaculate perhaps only once out of every two or three times that they make love. By delaying ejaculation, an older man may be able to become erect over and over again, continuing with intercourse and the pleasurable feelings it arouses.

Up to 60 percent of men in their seventies are still fertile, according to data from the Baltimore Longitudinal Study on Aging. In fact, there have been instances where fertility has continued into the nineties. A urologist can test for the presence of live sperm through a microscopic examination of semen. The important point here is that *fertility has no impact on erectile capacity*; even if a man loses his capacity to father children, his ability to have intercourse is not affected by loss of sperm production.

In general then, men do *not* lose their capacity to have erections and ejaculations as they age. The patterns of sexual activity of healthy men as they grow older tend to reflect earlier patterns in their lives, with the added factor of a somewhat slower physical response associated with aging. Problems that may occur, particularly erectile dysfunction, are caused by physical or psychological difficulties; *usually they are treatable.*

As for men's interest in sex or sexual desire, current studies indicate that desire appears to decline on average only slightly with age in healthy men. Further, sexual desire does not necessarily change even in those who experience an actual loss of erectile capacity or a change in orgasmic frequency. It is the amount of sexual activity itself, besides a decrease in ejaculatory amount, that does tend to decrease. Some speculate that this may be influenced by changes in the central nervous system that reduce the male's ability to translate visual sexual stimuli into physical arousal. Other factors may be disease processes under way but not yet obvious.

Finally, the unavailability of one's mate obviously has an impact upon the amount of sexual activity.

Ninety-one-year-old Henry, who lost his wife a number of years earlier, wrote to us:

> I have been "on the shelf," as they say, for the past four years—no more sex, just thinking about it, which is not sufficient. If I could find a lady friend who would accept a guy in a wheelchair, I might give it another try.

IS THERE A MALE MENOPAUSE?

Do men experience a period in life that is physically or psychologically comparable to a female's cessation of menstruation and loss of estrogen hormones? There is certainly no physical "menopause" or climacteric in men that is analogous to that in women, because hormone loss in men does not occur precipitously. (Actually, hormone loss in women occurs in spurts, never in a single, abrupt cessation.) Decreases in the male hormone testosterone take place very gradually with age. On average, men lose about 1 percent of their circulating testosterone concentration each year from age twenty-five on. However, this fluctuates widely from man to man. Some older men actually have testosterone levels identical with those in young men. Few men have specific physiological symptoms that can be traced directly to lowered testosterone levels. In a few uncommon cases, as with Perry, men do experience some physical problems.

Perry thought that his difficulties in obtaining an erection at the age of sixty-nine were a sign of "aging" and that it was all over for him when it came to sexual matters. He was more or less accepting of his fate. His wife, however, insisted on his seeing a doctor. She had to be incredibly persistent, for he was extremely reluctant to seek medical advice. Fortunately, it was discovered that his condition was among the rare instances of primary hypogonadism that constitutes low levels of testosterone. Through the artificial administration of testosterone, he was soon able to achieve an erection.

Distinct psychological symptoms are also rare when male hormone loss occurs, and can usually be accounted for by other circumstances in a man's life, such as his reactions to retirement, to aging in general, or to other stresses.

As research on male hormone levels becomes more sophisticated and reliable, it may eventually be possible to define a male climacteric, or as some have called it, "andropause" (other terms are "viropause" and "testopause"), particularly in light of some of the sexual changes that accompany male aging. However, it will be quite different from our concept of female menopause, with far less distinct and less predictable symptoms.

SEXUAL CHANGES—ARE THEY SIGNS OF AGING OR DISEASE?

We do not yet know whether all the physiological changes we have described in this chapter are "normal aging" processes or symptoms of preventable or reversible physical conditions. The fact that a man takes longer to achieve an erection as he gets older, or requires a longer period of time before an erection can occur again after the last sexual act, may possibly be related to reduced nutritive, oxygen, and blood supplies resulting from hardening of the arteries (arteriosclerosis), an extremely common condition. From a variety of studies we know that much of the physical change in other areas of men's lives that has been attributed to aging is in fact due to a variety of other factors, most notably the vascular diseases. The integrative systems of the body that link so many of its functions—the circulatory system, the endocrine (or hormonal) system, the central nervous system—all play a role in the decline of functioning when they are affected by diseases. We are only beginning to have some knowledge of the fundamentals of aging processes themselves: Is there a central-nervous-system pacemaker that dictates change? Are there reductions in the speed of reactions and in metabolism? Are there explanatory molecular and cellular changes? The answer to all of these is yes; it is in the details of how it all works that we remain bedeviled.

It is likely that in the future we will find that sexual

activity among older people actually improves as we increasingly separate out the diseases and psychological impairments of old age from the aging processes, and begin to prevent and treat them. Furthermore, if aging factors become more clear-cut and if agents that work to retard the process of aging are found, there will be still further changes in the sexual picture. What relatively healthy men and women need to remember, even under the limitations of our present knowledge about aging, is that sexual activity—to whatever degree and in whatever forms they want to express it—should continue to be possible, pleasurable, and beneficial. Those older people with fairly common chronic ailments can, in many cases, adapt their sexual desires so that they can find some form of satisfactory expression. Remember: Neither age nor in most cases infirmity automatically spells the end of sex.

CHAPTER 3

❧ ❧

COMMON MEDICAL
PROBLEMS AND HOW
THEY AFFECT
SEXUALITY

ILLNESS AND SEX

What happens to one's sexuality when illness strikes? An acute illness that is sudden and severe has an immediate effect. One's body and mind becomes totally involved in meeting the physical threat, and anxiety is strong until the crisis has passed and the full extent of the illness is known. Understandably, people in these circumstances have little or no energy and attention left for sexual feelings.

However, once the acute phase of an illness is over, most people return to sexuality, some slowly, others more quickly; but if recovery time is lengthy or if the illness results in a chronic condition which must be lived with, there can be problems. In this chapter we will discuss several of the more common conditions that may directly affect sexuality in people over sixty.

HEART DISEASE

Men from forty-five to sixty have heart disease at nearly three times the rate of women in this age group. After sixty the rates become more equal; many believe that postmenopausal women gradually become more vulnerable because of reductions in estrogen levels.

Sadly, heart (coronary) attacks lead many people to give up sex altogether under the assumption that it will endanger their lives—a phenomenon known as the fear of "death by orgasm." Such deaths are extremely rare. In an early 1990s study of over eight hundred men and women, Dr. James E. Muller of the Harvard Medical School and colleagues found *the chance of a heart attack during sex, among persons who had already had one, was only two in a million.* An earlier larger-scale study of more than 5,500 coronary deaths found that *less than 1 percent* were related to sex, with the majority of these involving extramarital relations (suggesting that stressful aspects associated with such affairs—i.e. guilt, anxiety, the need to hurry—may play a role). Thus, sexual activity poses extraordinarily little risk.

Yet recent studies show that many couples decrease or stop all sexual activity after a heart attack, often because their doctors haven't given them adequate advice. Fortunately, this picture is beginning to change as physicians remember to instruct and reassure patients on safe resumption of sexual activity and as patients become more forthright in asking for information. Studies show that the person who does resume sexual activity after a heart attack usually waits about sixteen weeks, with those who had the most active sex lives before a coronary resuming their sex lives the soonest. Many medical authorities believe that an *eight to fourteen-week waiting period* is an adequate amount of time before resuming sexual activity; of course, it all depends on the patient's desire, general fitness, and conditioning. Self-stimulation or mutual masturbation can be an alternative to sexual intercourse, and it can usually be started earlier. Some doctors propose a simple functional test to determine when it is safe to resume sex: *If you can walk briskly for three blocks without distress in the chest, pain, palpitations, or shortness of breath, you are usually well enough for sexual exertion.*

Sex *can* be carried out safely without sacrificing pleasure and quality. Studies tell us that, on the average, couples take ten to sixteen minutes for the sex act. The oxygen usage (or "cost") in sex is approximately equal to climbing one or two flights of stairs, walking rapidly at a rate of two to two and a half miles an hour, or completing many common occupational tasks. In average sexual activity the heart rate ranges from 90 to 160 beats a minute, which is the level for light to moderate physical activity. Systolic blood pressure (the upper reading, which reflects the contraction phase of the heart's action) may double, from 120 to over 240, and the respiratory rate rises from sixteen or eighteen to about sixty breaths a minute. These vital signs increase slightly more in men than in women, perhaps due in part to the frequent sexual position of the man on top. If the man is the one with the heart problem, conduct intercourse side by side or with the woman on top to reduce his exertion. These positions avoid the sapping of energy that occurs after a prolonged use of the arms and legs to support the body. Proper physical conditioning (usually a program of brisk walking and/or swimming) under a doctor's guidance and fitness trainers is useful, in part because such conditioning can lower the pulse-rate rise during sex.

Physical-fitness programs can enhance heart performance for a variety of activities, including sex. Isometric exercises (the exertion of effort against a stationary object like a wall), however, may be unwise for certain people because they cause pressure changes in the aorta, the major blood vessel from the heart, so be sure to check with your physician. If you have been physically inactive before undertaking an exercise program, ask your doctor to arrange special testing in which an electrocardiogram, or EKG (a tracing of the heart's electric currents that provides information regarding the heart's actions in health and disease), is taken while you engage in exercise at various intensities. An electromagnetic tape recording of your EKG during the sexual act can even be made in your own home. This is called Hellerstein's Sexercise Tolerance Test. Dr. H. E. Hellerstein and Dr. E. H. Friedman studied the sexual activity of men after recovery from an acute heart attack by monitoring sexual activities in the privacy of their patients' homes. They reported that if the men could perform exercise at levels of vigorous walking and other special activities without symptoms of abnormal pulse rate, blood pressure, or EKG changes, it was generally safe for them to resume sexual activity.

Some physicians warn, though, that such stress tests are not infallible. They can produce false alarms for healthy people, while in other cases coronary disease may not be detected. A medical and sexual history, the patient's report concerning any chest pain he or she may experience during exertion, and a resting EKG should all be part of the stress test.

Please remember that physical exercise leads to less likelihood of a heart attack. The sedentary person appears to be more prone to coronary attacks and less apt to survive the experience if one occurs. Too much food and alcohol before sexual intercourse can also place a strain on the heart. Of course, if the condition of the heart has deteriorated to the point that an attack is imminent, it may occur with any physical exertion, not merely sex. In fact, sexual intercourse may produce less increase in heart and respiratory rates than many everyday nonsexual activities.

It should also be realized that sexual arousal alone (without intercourse) affects the vital signs (although not as intensely as the sexual act itself). Failure to provide sexual release may prolong arousal, causing a psychological frustration that may produce some adverse physical effects.

Erectile problems can follow a heart attack for both physical and psychological reasons. A man may experience chest pain (angina pectoris) during various forms of exertion, including sex, that frightens him and thus prevents erection. To counteract this pain, take coronary dilators such as nitroglycerin (as discussed later, sildenafil citrate/Viagra should *never* be used with nitrates), prescribed by a physician, to improve circulation and reduce the pain just prior to sexual activity. A second common—and quite understandable—cause of erectile dysfunction is fear of inducing another coronary and risking death. This was the case with Frank.

Frank, age seventy-two, used to be amused by the fact that the French phrase for sexual orgasm is *le petite mort* (the little death). But it no longer seemed as funny after he had his heart attack and became obsessed with the thought that he might die from the exertion of sexual intercourse. It became virtually impossible for him to initiate sexual activity with his wife. She was puzzled and saddened by his remoteness, and finally insisted that they both see his heart doctor. Since Frank was too embarrassed to bring up the subject, she told the doctor what was wrong: Her husband was frightening himself into sexual inactivity. The doctor reassured both of them that Frank was in good enough physical condition to engage in any level of lovemaking. She demonstrated this by putting Frank on a treadmill and showing him the levels of physical exertion he could handle with no sign of overstress on his heart. Frank and his wife were greatly relieved and quickly returned to their usual patterns of sexuality.

Feeling depressed and anxious after a heart attack is common. You may also feel irritable and exhausted, and you might believe that your partner is no longer attracted to you. Conversely, your partner may become overly protective and fearful of upsetting you. In most cases, these are just normal reactions to what has been a tremendously frightening experience, and they will subside in time. If they do not, consider talking about these feelings with a physician or psychotherapist so that they do not harm your relationship or sex life.

Physicians, however, do not always advise their patients adequately on how and when to resume sexual activity after a heart attack. If you want to know more than your doctor has told you, it may be necessary to ask for specific information and directions, including a program of physical conditioning. Your partner also needs to be fully informed and counseled about any changes in lifestyle, and specifically lovemaking, that may be necessary. *Under most circumstances there is little reason to abstain from sex after a heart attack, and many reasons to continue!* You may experience pleasure, exhilaration, release of tension, mild exercise, and a sense of well-being. However, after resuming sexual activity, you should report any of the following occurrences to your doctor: (1) anginal pain occurring during or after sex; (2) palpitations continuing for fifteen minutes or more afterward; (3) unusual episodes of sleeplessness after sexual exertion; and (4) marked fatigue the next day.

To alleviate any potential stress during periods of lovemaking, it helps to: (1) have a familiar and considerate partner; (2) wait three hours or more after eating or drinking alcohol; (3) use a room with a moderate temperature; and (4) choose a relaxed time, such as the morning after a restful night. If you begin to feel strained or anxious during lovemaking, simply stop and breathe deeply for a few minutes before beginning again.

Episodes of congestive heart failure are also commonly called heart attacks. When they are compensated for by digitalis, diuretics, and diet, having sex is again an active possibility. However, it is advisable to wait two to three weeks after a congestive episode before having sex in order to make certain that the condition has stabilized.

Those with cardiac pacemakers need not give up sex unless the condition of their heart precludes such activity. But you should limit all forms of physical activity during the first two weeks following the implantation to allow for healing. The guidelines to follow will vary, based on your doctor's evaluation of the underlying cardiac condition.

CORONARY BYPASS SURGERY

Because of actual symptoms, the treatment of this disease, or the fear of sudden death from sexual activity, many people have some kind of sexual dysfunction by the time they have coronary bypass surgery. After the surgery, you must learn what level of activity you can undertake without stressing your chest bones. The sternum usually takes about three months to heal completely. Most of you will be advised to walk and move about very soon after the surgery. For those who fear the resumption of lovemaking, it may be reassuring to embark on exercise programs that improve heart capacity; this is what Ted, seventy-two, did after his bypass.

Ted had always been physically active: He was a runner, then a jogger, and more recently a fast walker. But his genetic background worked against him. He had a high level of cholesterol despite his excellent program of physical fitness and his diet, which stressed low fat and low cholesterol. His own view, which is shared by his doctor, is that had he not engaged in a vigorous physical and dietary program, he might not be alive today. Recently he had his first coronary bypass operation. It was his desire to continue his sex life that motivated him to make a quick return to his previous level of physical fitness. He visits the Pritikin Longevity Center in Florida annually to monitor his physical status, learn the latest diet and exercise techniques for his particular condition, and motivate himself to "stay on the program." As of this writing Ted has continued to stay healthy.

Many form a psychological dependence on taking nitroglycerin, a drug that alleviates chest pain, before having sex, even though surgery may have eliminated the need for it. To rid yourself of this dependency, obtain support from others who have successfully weaned themselves from nitroglycerin, or failing this, have your doctor prescribe a mild antianxiety medication for a brief time.

Those who require medications such as beta-blockers, which can decrease sexual desire and cause impotence, may be able to switch to other medications with fewer sexual side effects, such as calcium blockers like verapamil. Those with arrhythmias (irregular heartbeat) that do not require treatment need reassurance and perhaps a heart monitor (the Holter monitor) or a treadmill test to calm anxiety about sexual activity. In some cases antiarrhythmic drugs and beta-blockers cannot be avoided; if this happens to you, bear in mind that such drugs are life-protective, and if they interfere with your sexual desire and performance, you can and should concentrate on other forms of intimacy and physical pleasure.

In sum, then, many coronary bypass surgery patients can expect to return to a reasonable level of sexual activity. An exercise and nutritional program can improve your chances. *Short-term* treatment of anxiety and depression with the appropriate drugs can be helpful in leading toward the resumption of lovemaking, but in the long run you will find counseling, psychotherapy, and information about heart attacks to be more effective treatment methods.

HYPERTENSION

It is safe for most people with hypertension—high blood pressure—to have sex. (Many with hypertension have no significant impairment of heart function at all.) As a general rule, then, those with average to moderate hypertension need not restrict themselves sexually. You should, however, have your hypertension well controlled by diet, physical exercise, weight control, and, when appropriate, drug therapy. If you have very severe hypertension it may be best to modify your sexual activity; your doctor can best judge this.

Up to one-third of men with untreated hypertension are reported to have erectile dysfunction. This is not due to high blood pressure by itself, but rather, to associated atherosclerotic lesions. The effects of hypertension on female sexuality are less well studied. Sexual impairment can often be avoided by properly treating the hypertension. Weight loss if one is overweight (especially through the reduction of fat and sugar intake), regular exercise, reduction of cholesterol and triglyceride levels, limitation of salt to five grams or less a day, moderate use of alcohol, and no smoking are the first steps in treatment. Biofeedback therapies are also effective for some. If these do not bring your blood pressure down to acceptable levels, you will need medication. Such medication must be carefully chosen to avoid side effects of impaired sexual response (see page 148).

STROKE

Unless a stroke (cerebrovascular accident) causes severe trauma to the brain, sexual desire often continues; it is the physical performance that is more likely to be affected, especially in the earlier periods following the stroke. Men tend to have erectile and ejaculatory difficulty, while women may experience problems with vaginal lubrication.

However, strokes do not mean that all sexual activity must cease. Even if paralysis has occurred, appropriate sexual positions often can be found to compensate for it. The unaffected side of the body should be emphasized in lovemaking. When choosing a treatment plan, make sure that sexual rehabilitation is an important component of it. Use of bedboards and headboards can assist in positioning for sexual activity. It is also important to make note of the fact that sexual activity has *not* been found to be a factor in bringing on a stroke or in causing more damage to those who have had a stroke.

DIABETES

Sugar diabetes (diabetes mellitus) is a common occurrence in later life. Most men with diabetes are *not* impotent, but it *is* one of the few illnesses that can directly cause chronic potency problems in men. Erectile dysfunction occurs two to five times as often in diabetics as in the general population, and is often the first symptom of diabetes.

In most cases of diabetes-produced erectile dysfunction, sexual interest and desire are not affected, and the dysfunction itself may be reversible. There is some anecdotal evidence that when the diabetes is poorly controlled, upon proper regulation, erectile function will improve. This was the case with sixty-two-year-old Barry, who had his moderate diabetes under poor control.

Barry was a heavy smoker (two or more packs daily), and his travel schedule made good nutrition and proper exercise problematic. Barry suffered from both financial and marital troubles, and for him, all sexual activity had ceased. Luckily for Barry, his doctor insisted that Barry enter a treatment program where he was placed on a low-fat diet with carefully monitored amounts of physical exercise. Three weeks later his diabetes was under control and Barry had learned how to adapt his fitness program so that he could continue it while on business travel. And (this impressed him the most) his sexual capacity returned to him in full force.

There are a percentage of cases of diabetes in

which the erectile dysfunction is not reversible simply because the disease is controlled. When potency problems occur in well-controlled diabetes, sexual difficulties can become more complicated. And if you have been diabetic for a long time, the chances are greater that the erectile dysfunction will be difficult and sometimes even impossible to overcome. Further, problems may be exacerbated if there are concurrent endocrine problems such as a thyroid disorder. On a more positive note, however, the drug Viagra has recently been shown to be helpful for persons with chronic diabetes, and a trial period of Viagra is recommended even when the diabetic condition is severe (see page 121). If Viagra fails, prostaglandins (eg. Caverject, Muse) can still be effective.

With women it is more difficult to evaluate the effects of diabetes on sexuality, since women do not have an obvious physical indicator like erection. However, current research suggests that sexuality is affected far less by diabetes in women than in men.

CANCER

Although one out of every four Americans is expected to develop some form of cancer in his or her lifetime, survival rates are improving and many people who have had cancer go on to live normal lives. (Cancer generally develops in later life. Some 80 percent of all cancers occur after fifty and 50 percent after sixty-five.) However, the effects of cancer and its treatment can have a negative impact on sexual functioning. We will be discussing several examples in the next chapter. But because of the many different kinds of cancers and the complexity of cancer treatment, if the effects of cancer on sexuality are an issue for you, we recommend two excellent booklets by Leslie R. Schover, Ph.D., titled *Sexuality and Cancer: For the Woman Who Has Cancer and Her Partner* and *Sexuality and Cancer: For the Man Who Has Cancer and His Partner* (revised 2001), available from the American Cancer Society.

CHRONIC PROSTATITIS

Diminished sexual desire in men may be associated with chronic prostatitis. This disease is an inflammation of the prostate gland, a walnut-sized organ located just beneath the bladder in the male. It produces the milky lubricating fluid that transports sperm during sexual intercourse. You may experience pain in the perineal region (the area between the scrotum and the anus) and in the end of the penis on urination and ejaculation, and find that manual manipulation of the prostate causes tenderness. Treatment for such a condition includes antibiotics, warm sitz baths, and periodic gentle prostatic massage by a physician. Sexual desire usually returns after the pain lessens—especially when the pain after ejaculation is eliminated.

Many doctors believe that some cases of nonbacterial prostatitis are caused by both too frequent and too infrequent sex. The basis for some pain between the anus and the scrotum after ejaculation may be mild prostatitis; other causes are congestion due to excessive or lengthy preliminary sexual arousal, or an unsatisfying orgasm. However, a more common cause is infrequent sex, which results in congestion in the pelvic area. Treatment in these cases consists of more frequent ejaculation as well as gentle prostatic massage and warm sitz baths. Some believe that the practice of Kegel exercises (see pages 193) may help.

If you have chronic prostatitis, avoid excessive alcohol. Urinary retention can occasionally develop following sexual intercourse; this may be caused by the combination of a large fluid intake and the sedative effect of alcohol. If there is also some enlargement of the prostate without inflammation, excessive fluid intake, including alcohol, may lead to retention of urine.

ARTHRITIS

Arthritis, which comes in over one hundred forms, is a widespread condition that affects forty million Americans and strikes women twice as often as men. Rheumatoid arthritis, commonly beginning between ages twenty-five and fifty, and osteoarthritis, a later-life condition, are two major forms of arthritis and may cause pain during sexual activity. A third condition, fibromyalgia, involves muscles and attachments to bones. It is important to note that arthritis does not affect the sex organs themselves. Medications such as simple aspirin are used to reduce bone and joint pain. The Cox-2 inhibitors such as Celebrex and Vioxx are especially effective. It is reassuring to know that most drugs used to treat arthritis, except for corticosteroids, do not interfere with either sexual desire or sexual performance. You might also experiment with new sexual positions that do not aggravate pain in those joints that are sensitive. A well-established program of exercise, rest, and warm baths works wonders at reducing arthritic discomfort and facilitating sex. Indeed, much of the crippling effect of rheumatoid arthritis results from inactivity; a person tends to keep painful joints in comfortable positions, and they become stiffened, even "frozen." For information on exercise and other treatments, write for the free publication list published by the Arthritis Foundation, 122 East 42nd Street, New York, NY 10168, or call 212-984-8700. Several reprints dealing specifically with sexuality and arthritis are also available from the foundation.

Hip discomfort is perhaps the most frequent arthritic problem to affect sexual activity directly. Hip action during sex may be slowed down or made difficult because of pain or changes in the ability to move the hips. When the problem is severe, many choose surgical hip replacement, which may restore function, including that involved in sex. For less severe conditions, a range of therapies can be beneficial. Exercise, prescribed by your doctor, should include a full range of motion for the joints, strengthening and stretching of muscles, and engaging in the usual household and outside activities. You should also maintain an erect position when standing and walking, sit upright in a straight-backed chair, and rest in bed for short periods several times during the day. In general, rest or sleep in a straight position, flat on the back, using a small pillow under the head (a pillow under the knees can lead to stiff, bent knees).

The use of heat, both before undertaking an exercise program and prior to sex, relaxes any muscle spasms. Feel free to use various types of heat—heat lamps, heating pads, warm compresses, tub baths, showers, and paraffin baths. A daily tub bath with warm, not hot, water that lasts for no more than twenty minutes is excellent (longer baths can be fatiguing). A water bed and massage oils may enhance your comfort. Warming the bed with an electric blanket can be a great comfort. During lovemaking you may find that the side-by-side position—either face-to-face or back-to-front—is preferable, especially if you or your partner has tender areas and pain trigger points. As always, experiment until you find the positions that work best for you. Bear in mind that pillows can help in cushioning painful joints.

Timing can also be important. Some discover that pain and stiffness diminish or disappear completely at certain times of the day, so plan lovemaking for these times. Max and Molly, both in their early seventies, discovered the importance of this after retiring and settling in Florida. Their happiness at being retired and at having plenty of time for their personal relationship ran into snags, particularly with regard to their sex life. Molly has severe osteoarthritis, which gets worse at the end of the day. In particular, Molly has a great deal of discomfort in her hips. Together she and her husband consulted a sensitive and sympathetic internist, who encouraged them to take advantage of their retirement time and engage in lovemaking in the morning, after a good night's rest. This was the most pain-free time for Molly. Plus, it was suggested that they use the side-by-side sexual position, which puts less physical pressure on Molly. Even before beginning sexual activity, they found that a long, hot shower helped Molly relax physically. To further diminish her pain, she was advised to take aspirin and use pillows to cushion her hipbones. (Today a Cox-2 inhibitor might also be recommended.)

All of this enabled the couple to moderate and even eliminate Molly's arthritic pain. Furthermore, their time together became more intimate and tender than it had ever been at its best in their earlier years, because Molly was so touched by Max's concern for her.

Those who suffer from osteoarthritis, like Molly, will usually find morning to be the best part of the day, with discomfort increasing at the end of the day, while those with rheumatoid arthritis usually feel the greatest pain and stiffness in the morning. Be sure to ask your doctor to time pain or anti-inflammatory medications so they will be most effective at times when you are most likely to have sexual activity. A condition known as

Sjögren's syndrome occurs with some forms of arthritis and results in a decrease in body secretions. A lubricant such as KY Jelly will compensate for inadequate vaginal secretions.

Indeed, it may be physically beneficial for arthritis sufferers to engage in sex. Evidence suggests that regular sexual activity may produce some relief from the pain of rheumatoid arthritis for four to eight hours, probably because of adrenal gland production of the hormone cortisone and because of the physical activity involved. The body's release of endorphins, its natural pain relievers, during sexual activity and especially during orgasm may also be a factor. Finally, emotional stress can result from sexual dissatisfaction, and since stress worsens arthritis, satisfying sexual activity can be helpful in maintaining a healthy and pain-free body.

ASTHMA

Breathing problems can interfere with sexual activity just as with other forms of exercise. First of all, inform your doctor if you are having any breathing difficulties during physical exertion (shortness of breath, coughing, or wheezing), so that the cause can be determined and treated. If you typically take medication, such as a bronchodilator, before exercise, check with your doctor to see if you should do so prior to sexual activity. You may also want to experiment with sexual positions that do not put pressure on the chest. For severe asthma, sitting-up positions may be the most comfortable.

BACKACHE

Backache in the small of the back near the base of the spine is extremely common among older people. It is frequently caused by a generally inactive person's suddenly using the back muscles and placing strain on the back. In women the backache may also be traced to osteoporosis (postmenopausal thinning of the bones), which is related to the reduction in estrogen levels. Slipped discs and arthritis also cause backaches in both men and women.

Most backache sufferers need a firm mattress and bed board. A plywood board at least one-half inch thick and the same size as the mattress can be placed between the mattress and springs for extra support. Exercises for the back and the stomach are helpful for most forms of backache, but you should see your doctor and exercise therapist for instructions in your particular case. Walking, stationary bicycling, and swimming are frequently recommended. While slipped discs often respond well to exercise, sometimes they may require a period of bed rest; otherwise, as a last resort, surgery may be necessary. Those who suffer from arthritic backache should follow the program described above for arthritis.

Sexual activity itself is an excellent form of exercise

therapy for the back, stomach, and pelvic muscles, and if undertaken in a regular and reasonably vigorous manner, can help reduce back pain. A couple of aspirin (650 milligrams total) or one or two 500 milligram tablets of acetaminophen may help relieve pain, yet not mask your body's response to too much strain. During sex, you may find that the side position is the most comfortable if your back muscles are tender. Or you may prefer lying on your back, with your partner on top. Again, remember to support areas of discomfort with pillows. The standard "missionary posture," with the back-suffering person on top should be avoided. Also, do not arch backward or lie perfectly flat, since both of these positions put strain on the lower spine. Most cases of acute back pain disappear in four to eight weeks. Regular exercise, including appropriate sexual activity, can help insure that pain will not return.

ANEMIA

Anemia may develop insidiously following even a mild general or localized infection, or as a result of a poor diet. Tiredness, loss of appetite, and headaches are some of its early warning signs. Since anemia is a symptom of a number of diseases, as well as unrecognized blood loss, a comprehensive medical examination is needed. Follow-up treatment is extremely important. Often an improved diet with adequate vitamins and minerals is all that is necessary to restore both energy and sexual activity.

CHRONIC CYSTITIS AND URETHRITIS

Some women experience recurrent outbreaks of cystitis and urethritis following intercourse. The chief symptoms are severe pain and burning around the urethra. Yet the cause is often unclear, and if no organisms can be found in their urine, women are often told their problem is psychological. What this can lead to is outrage at the doctor, feelings of depression, continued pain, and a sense of hopelessness.

Do not give up even if you have to undergo a long diagnostic process by a gynecologist or a urologist until the cause or causes are found and corrected. Surgical correction, medications, diet, education on sexual techniques and positions, pain management, and interpersonal counseling are all possible avenues of treatment, depending on your physician's recommendation. And your sexual partner should be checked for possible untreated prostatitis. Plus, you must deal with the depression that usually accompanies chronic cystitis. Above all, your physician should persist in searching for the cause, and you should not be told it is all in your head. Take comfort in the fact that even long-standing cystitis can be evaluated and cured.

STRESS OR URGE INCONTINENCE

Nearly one woman in five over the age of forty will develop stress incontinence (caused by stretched pelvic muscles), a condition in which there is an involuntary seepage of urine because of a momentary inability to control the bladder. This happens particularly when you laugh, cough, bend, lift, engage in sex, or otherwise exert yourself. Urge incontinence is a sudden, painful urge to void (or no sensation at all) before you can get to a bathroom. Sexual dysfunction of various sorts has been reported in up to 50 percent of women with this condition. In fact, you might even experience dyspareunia, or painful intercourse. Stress incontinence is most frequently seen in women who have had a number of children and who might have unrepaired injuries following a birth, resulting in a relaxation of the uterine and bladder supports.

Obesity and estrogen deficiency can be strongly associated with the occurrence of incontinence. It is also seen in women who have had the uterus removed surgically (hysterectomy) or who have slack supporting tissues that may cause the bladder to protrude into the vagina (cystocele). Inserting a large tampon in the vagina, which gives support to the bladder, can sometimes provide temporary relief. To guard against toxic shock syndrome, do not leave the tampon in place for more than a few hours. Estrogen taken by mouth or applied locally in the form of a cream may help firm up the vaginal lining and thus reduce the irritation that may develop from the protruding bladder. You can also engage in specialized exercises, called Kegel exercises (described on page 193), to strengthen the muscles that support the bladder. Weight loss may have a positive impact on this condition. If the incontinence persists, you can purchase a wide variety of pads that provide hygiene security. Keeping bladder volume low by frequent voiding, especially before sexual or social encounters, is wise.

Biofeedback training can be helpful. However, the most severe cases of incontinence may require surgery to reposition the internal pelvic organs and tighten the muscles. Such surgery can be done under local or spinal anesthesia, and the success rate is very high.

A self-help and advocacy organization called the National Association for Incontinence (NAFI) can provide information and lists of resources. Write to NAFI, P.O. Box 8310, Spartanburg, SC 29305, and include a business-size self-addressed stamped envelope. NAFI will provide a list of its many helpful and informative publications on incontinence, as well as information about its quarterly newsletter, *Quality Care.* You may also wish to purchase NAFI's *Resource Guide of Continence Products and Services* as well as audio and videotapes.

The Simon Foundation for Continence, P.O. Box 835, Wilmette, IL 60091 (phone: 800-237-4666 or contact its Web site at www.simonfoundation.org), will provide information and a free copy of its quarterly newsletter, *The Informer.* The foundation published the first book for the layperson on the topic, *Managing Incontinence: A Guide to Living with the Loss of Bladder Control,* available at most local libraries or it can be purchased from the foundation.

Herniation, or prolapse of the uterus and of the rectum (rectocele), may occur alone or in association with prolapse of the bladder. In this case surgical treatment is usually effective. Stress incontinence is also occasionally seen in men following prostatectomy (see page 174).

In general, doctors agree that most stress or urge incontinence can be well controlled or even totally eliminated with the proper diagnosis and treatment. However, one of the greatest frustrations women voice is a lack of support and information from urologists, gynecologists, and other physicians when they report their incontinence problem. Be persistent and insist that your physician take effective action.

PARKINSON'S DISEASE

Parkinson's disease is a progressive nervous-system disorder of the later years marked by tremor, slowness of movement, partial facial paralysis, and peculiarity of posture and gait. Dementia can occur in 25 percent of patients in the course of their illness. Depression is commonly associated with Parkinson's disease and may lead to early potency problems in men and lack of sexual interest in both sexes. When there is advanced organic involvement, however, impotence may be physically connected with the disease. Those with Parkinson's disease who are treated with drugs such as levodopa (L-dopa) may show improved sexual performance, largely because of an increased sense of well-being and greater mobility. Levodopa is not an aphrodisiac, as some believe.

PEYRONIE'S DISEASE

This disorder, found in younger or middle-aged men, usually produces an upward bowing of the penis. A fibrous thickening of the covering of the corpora cavernosa of the penis produces the symptoms, but its cause is usually unknown. Sometimes the symptom disappears spontaneously. The results of nonsurgical treatment are unpredictable, and in fact are usually unsuccessful. One therapy involves taking potassium aminobenzoate (in the form of Potaba or Potaba Plus) for about six months. For some, the application of ultrasound to the fibrous areas of the penis in order to disrupt fibrous tissue has been successful, and this is especially true with those who have not had the problem for long. Surgical removal or incision of the plaque is often successful. Cortisone is sometimes effective, but it must be injected rather than taken orally. There is no evidence that vitamin E works. Counseling can help the patient adjust to the condition.

Intercourse can be painful in 50 percent of cases

and, if the penis is angled too far, impossible because penetration is precluded. However, in most cases of Peyronie's disease, sex can continue. This ailment is thought to be rare, but our own experience in talking with physicians and patients leads us to suspect that it may be more common than is believed.

PELVIC STEAL SYNDROME

The pelvic steal syndrome is an example of vascular impotence. In this condition the male loses his erection as soon as he enters his partner and begins pelvic thrusting. This impotence results from gravity's redirecting the blood supply from the penis to the muscles in the buttocks, which had been activated by the thrusting. To successfully overcome the pelvic steal syndrome, men should lie on their backs while making love, thus decreasing the demand for blood to the buttocks muscles and allowing it to flow to the penis. A side position may work as well.

CHRONIC RENAL DISEASE

Those with chronic renal disease experience a continuum of treatments that may end with renal dialysis or renal transplants. This can be a stressful disease and is often associated with depression and anxiety. Male chronic renal patients are often sterile and almost always have reduced levels of serum testosterone for unknown reasons. Other organic factors that affect one's sexuality may be present, although they have not been identified. Nonetheless, not all renal patients have sexual problems, and those who do may be treatable. Testosterone replacement is indicated not only for the treatment of impotence, but also to counteract muscle loss and osteoporosis. Treating the anxiety and the depression and engaging in marital counseling can also be helpful. Kidney transplants can often restore sexual capacity.

CHRONIC EMPHYSEMA AND BRONCHITIS

Chronic emphysema and bronchitis, which entail shortness of breath, often hinder physical activity, and that can include sex. The extent of the limitation depends on the severity of the disease. You'll find that resting at intervals and finding the least physically taxing ways to make love can help. Bronchodilators and oxygen use prior to sexual activity can also provide breathing relief.

HERNIA OR RUPTURE

A hernia or rupture is the protrusion of a part of the intestine through a gap or weak point in the muscular abdominal wall that contains it. The main complication to

avoid is strangulation, or a cutting off of the blood supply with the resulting death of tissue, which is a true surgical emergency. Straining of any kind, including
straining during sexual intercourse, can sometimes increase hernia symptoms such as pain and, rarely, induce
strangulation. Many surgeons recommend corrective
surgery early on, rather than waiting for an emergency
to arise.

A FINAL NOTE OF
REASSURANCE

If you have had to abstain from sex for a medical reason
for any length of time, some readjustment will be necessary when you resume sexual activity. Irregular or infrequent sexual stimulation can interfere with healthy
sexual functioning, adversely affecting potency in men
and lubrication, vaginal shape, and muscle tone in
women. These difficulties are likely to taper off as activity is resumed, so do not be discouraged by the initial
difficulties. When a sexual partner is not available or circumstances do not permit contact with a partner, both
men and women can protect much of their sexual capacity through regular self-stimulation (masturbation) if
this is acceptable and comfortable for them.

CHAPTER 4

✺〜✺

SEXUALLY TRANSMITTED DISEASES AND THEIR IMPACT ON OLDER PERSONS

ACQUIRED IMMUNE DEFICIENCY SYNDROME (AIDS)

AIDS is a condition caused by a virus called human immunodeficiency virus (HIV). The virus attacks the immune system, the body's "security force" that fights off infections. When the immune system breaks down, we lose this protection and can develop many serious, often deadly infections and cancers. These are called opportunistic infections because they take advantage of the body's weakened defenses. By far the greatest number of deaths associated with AIDS are caused by a virulent type of pneumonia known as Pneumocystis carinii pneumonia (PCP).

HIV can be transmitted through certain body fluids: blood, semen, vaginal secretions, and breast milk. While small amounts of the virus have been found in saliva, there have been no known cases of transmission by kissing or other contact with saliva, tears, or sweat. HIV enters the body through its mucous membranes (the lining of the rectum, the walls of the vagina, the inside of the mouth and throat). The virus cannot enter through the skin unless the skin is broken or cut and another person's body fluids enter the bloodstream. The virus also cannot be transmitted through the air by sneezing and coughing. This is why there is absolutely no danger in casual non-body-fluid contact with people who have HIV.

HIV has a long incubation period, which means that a person can have the virus for many years without knowing it and thus can unwittingly infect others. An individual is defined as having AIDS when he or she tests positive for HIV and displays evidence of serious damage to the immune system, such as pneumonia or another opportunistic infection. No one yet knows what percentage of people infected with HIV may develop AIDS, but at present it is thought that approximately 50 percent of those infected go on to develop AIDS within ten years. On the other hand, some people who have had the virus for at least fourteen years still show no symptoms of AIDS. Since the only reliable way of telling who is infected with the virus is through the antibody test, it is vitally important to understand and practice behavior that reduces the risk of transmission.

The two main vehicles for transmission are sexual intercourse and the sharing of needles with an infected person. To date in the United States 65 percent of AIDS cases involve homosexual or bisexual men, while 20 percent are intravenous (IV) drug users. While there has been much press about high-risk groups in the past, it is dangerous to allow this to lead you to think that if you are not homosexual or an intravenous drug user, you cannot become infected. A more accurate assessment of the situation is that *HIV does not recognize risk groups*. In Africa, for example, the overwhelming majority of AIDS cases are heterosexual men and women. And in the United States and elsewhere, the virus is more easily passed from a man to a woman than from a woman to a man. In the past, a small percentage of HIV transmission was caused by blood transfusions with HIV-infected blood. The risk of this route of infection is now very low; in 1985 a test was developed to screen blood for the presence of HIV.

Of all persons with active AIDS, 10 percent or more are over fifty years of age. One quarter of these are over sixty and 4 percent are over seventy. In the past, most of those who were older received HIV through blood transfusions; many have since died. Currently, the majority are gay men, although heterosexual transmission is increasing. AIDS is showing up more frequently in retirement communities. As of 1999, 78,000 people over fifty had developed AIDS, ten times more than a decade previously. Epidemiological studies show that those over age sixty diagnosed with HIV progress more rapidly to full-blown AIDS than those who are younger do, partly because they tend to be first detected at a late stage of infection. These older individuals also have a more severe set of opportunistic infections, possibly due to the combined effect of age and HIV on the production of T cells. (T cells are special cells in the bloodstream which, in a healthy person, attack the microbial agents of infections and thus are the building blocks of our immune system. HIV uses these T cells as factories for the production of more HIV, and over time destroys these cells, thus leaving the infected person with an impaired immune system.) Figures for rates of infection and those infected are currently changing. Decreasing rates of HIV infection among various communities of homosexual men prove that education and safer sex do work when they are taken seriously. However, in the year 2000 evidence of an upward trend in HIV in San Francisco suggests a relaxing of concern. Safer sex needs to be practiced by both men and women of all ages, heterosexual, bisexual, or homosexual.

To have safer sex and decrease your risk of infection, follow these procedures:

- Avoid any unprotected sexual contact that includes the exchange of body fluids (semen, blood, and perhaps saliva).
- Practice sexual monogamy (that is to say, have only one partner whose only partner is you—otherwise you are exposed to every person with whom your partner had unprotected sex). Unprotected sex (sex without a condom) with multiple partners greatly increases your risk of HIV infection.
- Use latex condoms in every sexual encounter. (If you have never used a condom before, you may want to send for *The Safer Sex Condom Guide for Men and Women*, published by GMHC, listed on page 100). Discard condoms whose shelf life has expired, since age can weaken them. Nonlatex condoms, such as those made of lambskin, do not effectively block the transmission of HIV. Also, spermicide-lubricated condoms have not been found to be more protective against disease than other condoms and in fact, have a shorter shelf life. (Ratings of condoms can be found in *Consumer Reports*, June 1999.) Glycerin or water-based lubricants, such as KY Jelly, may be

used to lubricate the outside of condoms and the female genital area. But never use oil-based lubricants (baby oil, mineral oil, petroleum jelly, and the like), since these can weaken the latex in condoms, causing tearing. Oil-based products may also foster vaginal infections.

- Avoid unprotected oral sex and/or deep oral kissing with a partner whose HIV status is unclear, since cuts or sores in the mouth can allow the virus to enter the bloodstream. The presence of genital herpes (in either party) triples the risk of HIV infection during sexual relations with an infected partner.
- Consider getting tested for HIV and other sexually transmitted diseases (STDs) if there is any chance that either you or your partner has been exposed to infection. A couple is considered safe from infection if both have tested negative and have been mutually monogamous for six months.

Many centers throughout the country offer information, support, testing, and help for people with AIDS or those who think they may be at risk. Most city public health clinics now offer free anonymous counseling and testing for HIV. The HIV antibody test can tell if your body has produced antibodies to HIV, so if you test positive, it means that you have been infected with the virus. While there is no cure for AIDS at this point, many treatments are available for those who test positive and these can delay—or even prevent—the onset of such life-threatening infections as PCP, mentioned above. The success of protease inhibitors has transformed AIDS into a chronic disease rather than a death sentence for those with access to this medication. In March 2001, the Centers for Disease Control and Prevention reported that the median survival time lengthened by four years (thus increasing the number of persons reaching fifty years of age and older). Furthermore, by greatly prolonging the lives of those infected, there is more time for better treatments to develop. It is critically important to be tested if you think you may be at risk. To find out about the testing center nearest you, call the National AIDS Hotline, on the next page. Here are some of the best sources of information about various aspects of AIDS:

AIDS EDUCATION AND INFORMATION RESOURCES

National Association on HIV over Fifty (NAHOF)
Southwest Boulevard Family Health Care
340 Southwest Boulevard
Kansas City, KS 66103
Contact NAHOF cochairperson, Jane P. Fowler,
    Phone: 816-421-5263
(Publishes a newsletter twice a year and offers

educational, prevention, service, and health-care programs for persons over age fifty affected by HIV. To subscribe call: 212-241-0719.)

National AIDS Clearinghouse (CDC National
    Prevention Information Network)
P.O. Box 6003
Rockville, MD 20849-6003
Phone: 1-800-458-5231
International Phone: 1-301-562-1098
(Provides information pamphlets and a materials
    catalog on request.)

National AIDS Hotline
Phone: 1-800-342-2437
TDD (for the hearing impaired): 1-800-243-7889
Spanish: 1-800-334-7432
(Provides educational pamphlets upon request and
    the names of other AIDS resources near you.)

Gay Men's Health Crisis (GMHC)
Publications/Education Department
119 West 24th Street
New York, NY 10011
Phone: 212-807-6655
TDD (for the hearing impaired): 212-645-7470
(Provides a wide range of services for men,
    women, and children affected by HIV and
    AIDS. Upon request will send the following

pamphlets: *AIDS Education Resources*; *HIV
and AIDS: The Basics*; *The Safer Sex Condom
Guide for Men and Women*; and *Medical
Answers about AIDS*.)

American Red Cross
AIDS Education Office
8111 Gate House Road
Falls Church, VA 22042
Phone: 703-206-7180
(Upon request, provides educational information
  on HIV and AIDS.)

AIDS Action Council
1906 Sunderland Place NW
Washington, DC 20009
Phone: 202-986-1300
(Provides information on policy and legislative
  issues relating to AIDS.)

Hispanic AIDS Forum
184 5th Ave. Floor 7
New York, NY 10012
Phone: 212-741-9797
(Provides information, referrals, and counseling to
  heterosexual, gay, and bisexual members of
  the Hispanic community. Telephone operators
  are bilingual.)

GENITAL HERPES

Caused by a virus known as herpes simplex 2, genital herpes affects as many as forty million Americans, and its incidence is increasing, with 300,000 to 500,000 new cases a year for the past few years. Genital herpes is moderately contagious, and is usually contracted through sexual contact. It is one of the rare sexually transmitted diseases that can also be contracted through sitting un-clothed in an infected place, especially in warm, moist environments such as hot tubs and whirlpools (although this is uncommon).

Symptoms appear in the form of itching and small, painful lesions in the genital or perirectal area four to seven days after sexual contact. Flulike symptoms may be present as well as general fatigue. These symptoms often disappear temporarily, only to recur. Most people with the active form of the disease have three or four flare-ups a year, each lasting several days to three weeks. The disease is most contagious during this time. Women with the disease may be at greater risk for cervical cancer.

If blisters or lesions do occur, they are treated with a cleansing salt solution. Secondary infections may be treated or avoided by use of oral sulfonamides. Though there is currently neither a cure nor a prevention for genital herpes, an antiviral drug, such as acyclovir (Zovi-rax), can prevent flare-ups of the disease; however, the long-term effects of such drugs are unknown. Flare-ups may recur if the medication is stopped. Acyclovir is available in IV, topical, and oral forms.

GONORRHEA

It is estimated that close to three million people in the United States are infected with gonorrhea annually. Men typically show obvious symptoms two to fourteen days after infection, with a tingling sensation in the urethra, and, shortly thereafter, pain during urination and a pus discharge from the penis. Some men may be asymptomatic for a period of time. In women, the disease is usually asymptomatic for weeks and even months. When symptoms do occur, they are in the form of a vaginal discharge and/or pain on urination, or frequency of urination.

Antibiotics are the usual treatment, although microbial resistance is developing. Both men and women are asked to refrain from sexual contact until they are cured, and all of those with whom they have had recent sexual contact should be traced and treated as well.

CHLAMYDIA

This may be the most common of all sexually transmitted diseases in the United States. It is often asymptomatic, especially in women. Any onset of unusual vaginal (women) or urethral (men) discharge should be cause for concern. Additional symptoms include pain on urination in men and frequent urination and painful intercourse in women. Anyone experiencing these symptoms should be tested to rule out other sexually transmitted diseases. Once a diagnosis of chlamydia is made, it is easily treated with antibiotics such as tetracycline. If left untreated, chlamydia can cause urethral infections and inflamed testes in men and inflammation of the Fallopian tubes in women.

SYPHILIS

Syphilis is caused by an infectious organism that enters the lymph glands. If untreated, the disease can unfold over a period of years in three stages, the last of which is a fatal infection of the heart, brain, or other organ. Fortunately, nearly all cases are now detected in the primary stage. Lesions (chancres or sores) appear about four weeks after infection, or skin rashes in six to eight weeks. Penicillin is the antibiotic treatment of choice for all three stages. Sexual activity must stop during treatment, and all with whom you have had sexual contact in the preceding three to twelve months should be identified and treated. You need to be retested by your doctor until all traces of the disease have disappeared. A rising incidence of syphilis in recent years was principally associated with drug addiction and AIDS. However, by the year 2000, the incidence of syphilis was falling significantly in the United States. Nonetheless, it is still a concern for the general population.

HEPATITIS B

Most people don't realize that hepatitis B is a serious virus that is either sexually transmitted or spread through contact with infected blood or other body fluids. It can cause severe liver damage and may result in chronic hepatitis or even death from related illnesses. An estimated 200,000 Americans are infected with hepatitis B each year, and an estimated 5,000 die of complications from the disease. Hepatitis B is the *only* sexually transmitted virus preventable by vaccine. Any person, regardless of age, who is sexually active outside of a strictly monogamous relationship should receive one of the two vaccines now available. See your physician for advice and access to the vaccines.

In Summary

The early detection and treatment that have been—and essentially still are—the solution for gonorrhea, syphilis, and most recently chlamydia, as well as the vaccines now available to prevent hepatitis B, are inapplicable to diseases such as genital herpes and especially AIDS. The sole protection against these currently incurable diseases is behavior changes that prevent their contraction in the first place. We outlined recommended sexual behaviors to lessen the risk of exposure to AIDS, especially the avoidance of unprotected sexual activity. In the meantime, continued research is necessary to learn how to control this dangerous and deadly public health threat.

CHAPTER 5

❧❧

ERECTILE DYSFUNCTION (IMPOTENCE)

WHAT IS ERECTILE DYSFUNCTION?

Erectile dysfunction (ED), often referred to as "impotence," is the loss of a man's ability to obtain an erection sufficient to achieve or maintain sexual intercourse. The term "impotence" is actually an inexact way to describe what many men experience. It is rare for men to totally lose the capacity for at least *some* degree of erection; however, less than a full erection can interfere with full sexual expression. The severity of the impotence ranges from being incapable of a total erection some of the time to being incapable most or all of the time. Erectile dysfunction also refers to the inability to sustain an erection even if one is initially able to have one.

It is estimated that anywhere from twenty to thirty million American men (about 70 percent are over fifty years of age) suffer from chronic erection problems, with perhaps ten million others having less severe dysfunction. This is *not* part of the normal physical process of growing older, even though such problems may increase with age, due to physical illness and other causes. It is estimated that only about 5 to 10 percent of men with erectile dysfunction seek help. If erectile problems occur regularly, you should investigate the cause or causes and treat the condition; do not let your physician or anyone else discourage you from seeking help. According to many experts, up to 90 percent of cases can be improved or even reversed with proper diagnosis and treatment. Therefore a man with erectile dysfunction *must* be examined medically to determine whether or not a physical condition is acting as a partial or complete cause of this condition.

WHAT PRODUCES AN ERECTION?

The physiology and psychology of getting and maintaining an erection are complicated and are based on reflexes rather than a man's conscious control. Two sets of messages—stimulation of the penis through touch and/or stimulation of the brain through erotic thoughts triggered by sights, smells, sounds, memories, or fantasies—are sent to nerve centers in the spinal cord. These nerve centers then convey messages to the penile blood vessels, causing them to enlarge and fill with blood (engorge), creating an erection. At the same time, the blood is prevented from leaving or leaking out of the penis. Testosterone and chemicals known as neurotransmitters (principally, nitric oxide) play an important role. (For those with a medical or scientific background, see an excellent review on erectile dysfunction by Tom F. Lue in *The New England Journal of Medicine*, 342: 1802–1813, June 15, 2000.) In adolescents and very young men, mental stimulation is often enough to produce an erection. However, most men in their late forties and thereafter will often find that they need tactile (either manual or oral) stimulation of the penis, in addition to erotic visual stimuli, and/or erotic thoughts and mood before an erection occurs. One man in his late sixties who spoke to us reported on the success of this route: "For thirty-six years my wife and I enjoyed an active sex life. But then I began to have difficulty getting an erection. My wife felt she was no longer sexually attractive, and I thought I was a failure. We went to a sex counselor, who told us that in addition to our usual patterns of lovemaking, I now needed physical stimulation to get an erection. We started to do this regularly, with my wife stimulating me by hand prior to intercourse. As a result, our sex life has greatly improved. And as an added plus, once my penis is erect, it stays hard much longer."

At What Age Are Erection Problems Likely to Occur?

There has been little reliable scientific information concerning the actual experience of erectile difficulties as men grow older. Kinsey documented a decline in potency up until the age of fifty, but his sample over fifty was too small to draw conclusions. Duke University and the Gerontology Research Center of the National Institute on Aging in Baltimore have found a general pattern of decline as well. About 25 percent of men who are sixty-five and older have a significant degree of erectile dysfunction, as well as 50 percent of men over eighty. There is, however, much individual variation. Indeed, a significant proportion of men had stable and even rising patterns of sexual activity with age. For our purposes here, it is clear that erection problems do increase with age (due to illness or other causes—but *not* due to physical aging itself); however, such problems are not inevitable, nor are they by any means always permanent.

It is important to point out the critical importance of a man's emotional relationship to his partner. Intimacy and affection can transform a mundane or flawed physical sexual encounter into one characterized by tenderness and love—compensating for and at times even completely overcoming imperfect physiological functioning.

THE MIND-BODY ISSUE IN ERECTILE DYSFUNCTION

It has long been generally (but falsely) accepted that at least 90 percent of erectile dysfunction in men over sixty was psychologically based, with only about 10 percent physiologically caused. These figures, quoted since the 1920s, can be traced back to the book *Impotence in the Male*, by one of Freud's colleagues, William Stekel.

William Masters and Virginia Johnson, the pioneer sex researchers, arrived at the same conclusions in their laboratory studies of older men, and some psychotherapists and sex counselors have continued to promulgate these beliefs. The proportion of psychologically based potency problems among men forty to sixty had previously been estimated to be even higher, at 95 percent. However, more effective diagnostic techniques and a growing understanding of the physiology of erectile dysfunction are starting to change those views. In the last few years, biomedical researchers, using a variety of more sophisticated measurements and advanced techniques, including sleep studies, have begun to demonstrate that erectile difficulties may have a much higher physiological component, perhaps involving 80 to 90 percent of all cases of potency problems, *regardless* of age. The figure is highest for older men, especially those with vascular conditions.

As a general rule, if the onset of erectile dysfunction is sudden and the course is intermittent, the cause is probably psychological, such as recent widowhood, and other intense emotional stress. If the onset is slow—over a period of six months to a year—and the course chronic, the cause is much more likely to be physical.

In this book, we have made an artificial division between physically-based and psychologically-based erectile dysfunction, simply to facilitate our discussion. In truth the two are usually intermixed, although there is often a greater emphasis in one direction or another. The psychological aspects of erectile dysfunction are discussed in later chapters.

MAJOR CAUSES OF PHYSICALLY-BASED ERECTILE DYSFUNCTION

In a significant number of cases of erectile dysfunction, a physical illness has probably gone undetected or at least a mixed diagnosis involving physical as well as emotional components has been overlooked. This helps to explain the estimated 60 percent or higher failure rate from using psychotherapy alone to treat potency problems. According to one classification, the major causes of primarily physically-based ED are listed in order of occurrence below:

PHYSICAL PROBLEMS

Diabetes mellitus
Vascular insufficiency (arteriosclerosis, hypertension, antihypertensive medications [beta blocker agents])

Radical surgery (prostatectomies, colostomies, cystectomies, etc.)

Trauma (spinal cord injuries, pelvic fractures, etc.)

Hypogonadism and other endocrine disorders

Multiple sclerosis

Peyronie's disease (fibrous cavernitis)

Side effects from medications and other drugs (estrogens, anticholinergic drugs, excessive tranquilizers, antidepressants, antihypertensive agents, opiates, alcohol, nicotine, etc.)

Under ideal circumstances, the diagnosis of sexual dysfunction should be multidisciplinary, potentially involving relevant specialists in internal medicine, endocrinology, neurology, urology, radiology, vascular therapy, psychiatry, psychotherapy, and sex therapy. Insurance plans, including Medicare, will cover a portion of the diagnostic costs as well as some forms of treatment. Any evaluation and treatment should take into account your partner as well. To save both time and money, though, make sure that initial treatment efforts focus on adjusting the dosage of any drug you are taking that is associated with erectile dysfunction or changing to a similar drug without the adverse side effect of erectile problems. Do not, however, stop taking a medicine you think may be causing the problem without speaking with your physician. You should also not be surprised to find yourself encouraged to undertake changes in your lifestyle, including improving your diet, quitting smoking, reducing your alcohol consumption, losing weight, and exercising.

And what diagnostic procedures can you expect to undergo? They may require any or all of the following:

- A thorough history, including your past sex life, possible psychiatric and psychological contributors to erectile dysfunction, review of alcohol and drug use, and past or present illnesses.
- A physical examination.
- A sleep study, which monitors your erections during sleep. A portable home monitor, called a RigiScan, is a simple and inexpensive method of testing for erections in your own home. Minimal erections or the absence of erections during sleep strongly suggests, but does not definitely prove, an organic basis for erectile dysfunction. For information on clinics that conduct such studies, contact the American Academy of Sleep Medicine, 6301 Bandel Road, Rochester, MN 55901, Phone: 507-287-6006.
- Testing of erectile functioning through other methods. This includes visual stimulation, the use of a vibrator, or a prostaglandin-E-1 (PGE-1) injection alone or in combination

with another medication called phentolamine directly into the penis. These penile injections occasionally produce an erection lasting more than an hour in those who are sexually excited *and* physiologically normal. (This can be very effective psychologically, for it demonstrates to an individual with psychological-based erectile dysfunction that he *can* have an erection.) Penile blood flow measurements may be useful, as well as glucose tolerance tests to rule diabetes in or out. Indeed, there should be an endocrinological screening to rule out various hormonal dysfunctions such as thyroid, testosterone, and prolactin abnormalities. It should also measure your level of cholesterol, triglycerides, LDL, and HDL.

While pudendal arteriography (injecting a special dye into the main artery that supplies the penis to study blood flow) can accurately assess penile arterial disease, it is quite expensive and physically invasive. You and your doctor may choose to estimate penile blood flow through penile duplex ultrasound using a vasodilator, such as PGE-1.

TREATMENT FOR ERECTILE DYSFUNCTION

The first step in the treatment of erectile dysfunction is attention to any underlying medical disease, physical disability, or health habits such as alcohol abuse, smoking, and various prescription, over-the-counter, and illegal drugs that may be contributing to sexual problems. Recommendations for exercise and nutritional changes may also be warranted since both obese men and sedentary men have higher rates of ED. However, when dysfunction persists after the above measures are taken, specific treatments are available.

TESTOSTERONE

Male hormone therapy (sex-steroid replacement with testosterone) has little known permanent beneficial effect on the sexual problems of older men unless there is definitely a proven testicular deficiency in the production of male hormones—known as hypogonadism. It is estimated that only about 5 percent of men have low serum testosterone levels, but 15 to 20 percent have low bioavailable serum testosterone levels, requiring testosterone replacement. Testosterone levels can be determined by a simple blood test, although measurement of bioavailable levels may have to be done in university hospital laboratories or other specialized settings. Levels vary considerably. For example, a seventy-five-year-old man on average has testosterone blood levels that are 35 percent lower than in younger men. However, one quarter of all seventy-five-year-olds have levels similar to those of younger men. Even when levels are lower, they are still sufficient for normal sexual response in most older men.

Testosterone's primary function in sexuality is to maintain the libido or sex drive. It has been shown to have little direct effect on the capacity for erections. Testosterone is administered in pills (no longer recommended because of connections with liver toxicity), intramuscular injections (which can be painful and don't always provide constant blood levels of testosterone although they cost much less than other methods), testosterone patches (Androderm and Testoderm patches are worn on the scrotum or elsewhere and can cause skin irritations), and AndroGel, a lotion designed to be rubbed daily on the shoulders, upper arms, and/or abdomen. It is absorbed into the bloodstream through the skin. Although approved for men by the FDA in February 2000, it has not been approved for use in women. It is an expensive treatment—$300 for a two-month supply. Hands should be thoroughly washed after applying AndroGel and the treated skin should be covered once AndroGel dries. If another person has contact with the gel (including skin-to-skin contact during sexual activity), the area of contact should be washed with soap and water.

Men who do not have hypogonadism are discouraged from using testosterone. Any benefit from testosterone treatments may show up in three to four weeks, but even in those who do appear to respond, the improvement may be short-lived. The beneficial effects do not tend to be maintained indefinitely except in those with clear-cut hormone deficiencies. (Note: Viagra can be used together with testosterone replacement therapy.) There may also be side effects, such as fluid retention, a thickening of the blood, breast formation, hair loss, and possibly a lowering of "good" HDL cholesterol. Testosterone is definitely not indicated if prostate cancer is already present. All men should have a digital rectal exam and a prostate-specific antigen (PSA) test to try to rule out cancer before considering testosterone supplementation.

VIAGRA (SILDENAFIL CITRATE)

Viagra has had a dramatic effect on the treatment of erectile dysfunction. In 1992, five years before the appearance of Viagra, a million American men received pharmacotherapy in the form of self-injections, 30,000 used vacuum systems, 20,000 had penile implants, and 1,500 had been subject to vascular surgical repair. Most treatment was carried out by urologists and other medical specialists and was characterized by physical invasiveness. By 1998, sildenafil citrate under the brand name of Viagra entered the market as the first successful oral medication for erectile dysfunction. It caused an overnight sensation. Former U.S. Senator and presidential nominee Bob Dole became one of its spokespersons, opening up a nationwide dialogue on the seldom discussed topic of male impotence. As of 2001, some ten million men in the United States had received Viagra prescriptions and more than 30 million prescriptions had been dispensed, this time largely by primary care doctors (in 90 percent of instances) and a lesser number of cardiologists and pulmonary doctors rather than specialists in male dysfunction. Urologists became the last rather than the first line of defense, their services reserved for complicated situations such as those in which men failed to respond to Viagra.

HOW DOES VIAGRA WORK?

Viagra relaxes blood vessels and creates greater blood flow, thereby enabling men to achieve erections. The accompanying increase in nitric oxide in the penis is a critical factor.

Viagra is not an aphrodisiac (except through the power of suggestion) and has no physiological effect on sexual desire. Therefore, its drug action will not enhance sexual performance unless a man is having true physically-based erectile difficulties. It will also not work unless a man is mentally/emotionally aroused in addition to taking the drug.

It requires about an hour to become effective and although it remains in the body for up to eight hours, the best erectile effects are achieved in the first four hours. Most physicians recommend no more than one pill a day.

WHO CAN BE HELPED BY VIAGRA?

The success rate is 60 to 70 percent or more among those taking Viagra, although rates vary substantially, depending on the type and severity of underlying medical conditions. Viagra has been found to be effective for men with Type I and Type II diabetes, spinal cord injury, multiple sclerosis, heart disease (except for those taking nitrates or in certain cases of advanced heart disease with severe atherosclerosis), chronic renal failure, Parkinson's disease, spina bifida, hypertension, depression, anxiety, and those who have had prostate cancer treatment or have received transplants.

To improve chances of success, patients with medical risk factors must take steps to reduce those risks, preferably before using Viagra (ideally two months prior to use). This includes stopping smoking, decreasing alcohol intake, diagnosing and treating new diabetes or hypertension, and treating hyperlipidemia with elevated LDL.

Men may have a lessened response or no response if they have had nonnerve-sparing radical prostatectomies, poorly controlled diabetes, or multiple diabetic complications. However, Viagra should be tried, as it *may* help. In some cases of nerve damage, erection may be possible but not orgasm and ejaculation.

Spokespersons for Pfizer indicate that there is no upper-age limit for Viagra use. Men up to the age of ninety were included in the original clinical trials.

Although most patients respond after one to two doses, it may take up to seven to eight doses (over as many days) to achieve success. About one third of users do not achieve an erection sufficient for penetration. This is especially true for men who have had radical prostate cancer surgery. However, even patients who have had bypass surgery or angioplasty may take Viagra as long as their blood flow remains unobstructed.

Viagra may help with the negative sexual effects of many psychoactive medications, including the selective serotonin reuptake inhibitors (SSRIs). The recommendation is to first control the depression with medication, then add Viagra to counter the sexual side effects.

Men with "performance anxiety" or other psychological-based erectile problems have been reported cured just by having Viagra in their medicine cabinets—a sort of psychological safety net in case they need it.

As a result of coming to their physician about possible Viagra use, a significant number of men have also been diagnosed with untreated diabetes, high blood pressure, and heart disease and began receiving treatment. Thus, Viagra proved to be a lure enabling them to receive critical medical evaluation and care for underlying diseases.

WHO SHOULD NOT TAKE VIAGRA?

Men taking nitrates for heart pain should not take Viagra because of the danger of a fatal drop in blood pressure that could trigger a heart attack. Early clinical trials by Pfizer did not include severely ill men, especially those with heart disease. By January 1999, the FDA confirmed 130 deaths among Viagra users, 77 of them from coronary problems. Some but not all of these deaths occurred among men who were also taking nitrates. The FDA also reported that hundreds of others suffered nonfatal heart attacks, strokes, and other untoward incidents. Although it was unclear how many of these were related to Viagra rather than to already present diseases that would have caused the incidents in any case, after the FDA's findings Pfizer's response was to issue stronger warnings about contraindications.

Viagra may also be contraindicated for some persons with blocked or constricted arteries, although several recent studies suggest cardiac risk may be minimal. Nonetheless, patients with severe coronary heart disease should be evaluated as to the risks and benefits of sexual activity. Some physicians now insist on treadmill and other tests in order to gauge heart fitness.

There is no controlled clinical data on Viagra's safety for patients with heart attack, stroke, or severe arrhythmia within the past six months. This also is true for patients with resting hypo- or hypertension and retinitis pigmentosa.

Angina or chest pain, even without use of nitrates, is a contraindication to Viagra use.

Emergency-room personnel must be aware of Viagra use in men who arrive with possible heart attacks. It is critically important that patients or their friends or family members inform physicians, so as to avoid administering nitrates.

Patients should be able to demonstrate sufficient exercise capacity to have sex safely. If they do not, a program of regular exercise should be added first. It may also be advisable to start sexual activity on a measured basis to judge physical tolerance.

Viagra should not be used with amyl nitrate (poppers). Gay men in particular should be aware of this danger.

Viagra should not be used with other treatments for erectile dysfunction, such as penile injections, implants, or vacuum pumps since such combination therapy has not been tested.

WHAT ARE THE DOSAGES?

Viagra is administered once a day in pills containing 25 milligrams, 50 milligrams, or 100 milligrams of sidenafil. Men, including those who are older, usually begin at 50 milligrams. The highest dose of 100 milligrams is used only when 50 milligrams prove ineffective.

TIPS ON HOW VIAGRA SHOULD BE TAKEN

Take Viagra on an empty stomach or at least not after a high-fat meal which will delay the drug's onset. Avoid smoking and drinking heavily. Be well rested. Allow at least forty-five minutes for the drug to be absorbed. Remember that it works for three to four hours.

A relaxed setting is important. Some men may feel more comfortable taking Viagra for the first time while masturbating, thus eliminating a feeling of pressure for performance. However, in general, partner involvement is crucial, including romance, foreplay, and sensuality. Viagra will not work without erotic stimulation.

WHAT ARE THE SIDE EFFECTS?

Possible side effects include headache, flushing, stomach upset, nasal congestion, transient increased sensitivity to light, and color vision disturbance (seeing blue). Side effects are highest in those taking the highest doses. Most side effects are mild to moderate, and self-limited in the length of time they persist. Any chest pains, nausea, or dizziness should be reported to the prescribing doctor and Viagra use should be stopped.

OTHER POSSIBLE COMPLICATIONS WITH VIAGRA

Increased sexual activity may bring out hidden relationship problems that were previously dormant when sexual contact was limited or nonexistent. These issues then require attention.

A frequent complaint for female partners is an increase in "honeymoon cystitis," especially in those in the age range of fifty-five to seventy-five who may not have had intercourse for some time or who have vaginal dryness. (Using vaginal lubricants and drinking a cup of water shortly before and after intercourse can help. If cystitis persists, antibiotics may be necessary.)

Viagra can be purchased over the Internet without proper medical oversight. The National Association of Boards of Pharmacy, the FDA, and state attorneys general are finding it difficult to locate and prosecute dangerous on-line pharmacies. This is problematic for a number of reasons: 1) Erectile dysfunction is frequently a symptom of underlying diseases which should be medically diagnosed and treated before other remedies are sought. 2) Those who take nitrates may inadvertently expose themselves to dangerous drug interactions with Viagra. 3) Youngsters experimenting on drugs can obtain Viagra by disguising their ages and physical conditions.

The high cost per pill ($8 to $10) can be a detriment. In addition, a number of insurance companies will not reimburse for "recreational" drugs unless true erectile problems can be medically demonstrated. When Viagra is covered, insurance companies and HMOs may limit the number of pills per month. Medicare does not cover any outpatient prescription medications.

Some men with erection difficulties prefer the nearly immediate and long-lasting erection resulting from injections (described later) than the hour's wait before Viagra takes effect.

Priapism can occur in some men, namely an erection that does not subside and requires emergency treatment. *(An erection lasting for more than four hours is considered a medical emergency.)*

OTHER ORAL DRUGS FOR ERECTILE DYSFUNCTION

Apomorphine (Uprima), originally used for Parkinson's disease and in emergency rooms as an emetic (to induce vomiting), is a stimulant that increases levels of the brain chemical dopamine, thereby causing erections. It has been considered a possible major rival to Viagra. Troublesome side effects have included vomiting (in more than 15 percent of patients), nausea, and fainting. Uprima is currently in phase III clinical trials, with its researchers hoping for FDA approval, although prospects look dim. *Vasomax*, a drug aimed at increasing penile blood flow, has not been approved in the United States. Clinical trials have been halted because of problems with the drug in test animals. *Trazadone*, an antidepressant medication, has not been found to be useful. *Oral phentolamine* has been reported to improve erectile function but may, in rare cases, cause potentially lethal hypotension. It does not have FDA approval for use in sexual dysfunction.

A sizable number of other drugs for both men and women are currently in various stages of clinical trials. All are aiming at the huge sexual dysfunction market currently dominated by Viagra. Some of the drug companies involved are Senetek (developing a drug called Invicorp for penile injection), Harvard Scientific (a pellet/plunger similar to MUSE [see p. 131], but easier to use), ICOS (a Viagra-like pill called IC351, said to have fewer side effects than Viagra), and Palatin Technologies (a drug called Erectide, an erection drug injected elsewhere than the penis). Cialis (by Eli Lilly and Icos) and Vardenafil (by Bayer AG) are similar to Viagra, with possibly fewer side effects, quicker action, and longer effects. Both are awaiting FDA approval.

SELF-INJECTED DRUG THERAPY

If one can become comfortable with the thought of self-injection of vasoactive compounds (called intracavernous pharmacotherapy) directly into the shaft of the penis, this treatment can be valuable in helping produce an erection. However, the "cringe" factor surrounding the thought of this procedure can be difficult to overcome. In reality, the extremely fine, small-gauge needles are relatively painless. In such a treatment you must follow strict sterile procedures, and there should be long-term follow-up.

In the past the most popular substance for this kind of self-injection was a mixture of papaverine hydrochloride and phentolamine. However, the U.S. Food and Drug Administration has not officially approved using papaverine for this purpose, and its manufacturer, Eli Lilly, states that the drug "is not indicated for the treatment of impotence by intracorporeal injection." Nonetheless, many urologists use it for this purpose, and the American Urological Association recognizes its value. Patients who have mild to moderate vascular-based erectile problems are usually the best candidates for this type of treatment. (Ordinarily, self-injection therapy is not effective in the presence of severe vascular disease.)

Prostaglandin-E-1 (PGE-1) or alprostadil (Caverject or Edex)—another drug that can be self-injected directly into the penis—has now been found to be effective in many patients, even those who do not respond to papaverine. Due to its few side effects, many urologists are currently using this drug alone or in combination with papaverine or phentolamine or both (termed a "trimix"). An erection occurs in several minutes and lasts for sixty minutes or so. High rates of satisfaction are reported with this drug's use. It is especially helpful in patients with diabetes, surgery, and injury.

Long-term injection therapy can eventually prove to be a problem, particularly when it comes to high doses of papaverine. The quality of the erections produced sometimes declines over time. And occasionally, priapism—sustained erection lasting longer than four hours—can occur. (These prolonged erections must be reversed. This can be done medically either by aspiration of a small amount of blood or by injecting dilute epinephrine or phenylephrine.) Lastly, if not used properly, there can be intense scarring of the penis, which may make implantation of a prosthesis, if it is needed later, difficult or even impossible.

In spite of all these difficulties, some find the self-injections invaluable and become quite accustomed to them, just as diabetics become used to insulin injections. Self-injection works best in those whose erection difficulties are caused by nerve damage (as a result of spinal cord injury, lumbar disc disease, radical pelvic surgery, multiple sclerosis, or juvenile onset diabetes) and in those affected by poor circulation. However, some hypertensive individuals experienced prolonged erections as a side effect of injecting combined papaverine hydrochloride and phentolamine mesylate into the penis. Men who experience psychogenic erectile dysfunction can also use the self-injection method temporarily.

Muse is another form of alprostadil, but instead of being injected with a needle, it is released through a small plunger which is inserted about an inch into the urethra. Speed and length of erection are similar to Caverject. Priapism and scarring of the penis are minimal. However, it is less effective than self-injected medications.

EXTERNAL VACUUM DEVICES

When Viagra or other treatments don't work or are contraindicated, some men use external vacuum devices (EVDs) to obtain and maintain erections. For this procedure, you fit a plastic-cylinder vacuum device over the limp penis, attach a piece of plastic tubing to an opening in the end of the device, and then suck the air out with a syringe, a pump, or your mouth. Battery-driven devices are also available. This produces a gentle vacuum that encourages blood flow into the penis, creating an erection. Once a full erection occurs, a wide rubber band, or constriction ring (they are available in different sizes), stored on the end of the cylinder nearest the base of the penis, is slipped around the penis's base to retain the blood, thus maintaining the erection. All in all, the device and the procedure for using it are fairly cumbersome. Furthermore, the constriction band should only be left on for thirty to forty minutes. But according to Dr. E. Douglas Whitehead, a urologist and director of the Association for Male Sexual Dysfunction in New York City, EVDs have proven to be up to 80 percent successful in creating and maintaining an erection sufficient for the duration of intercourse. Others estimate success in the 30 to 50 percent range. Compared to an implant, this method is much less expensive, and does not permanently alter the penis since no surgery is involved.

You do need a physician's prescription to obtain an EVD. And bear in mind that its long-term safety and effectiveness are still being evaluated. Men on anticoagulant therapy or those who have blood abnormalities should not use EVDs. Also, a small proportion of men report that their ejaculation is blocked and this may result in pain. But in general, most find that an orgasm is both possible and pleasurable, and that their partner's satisfaction is also high, especially when their relationship is otherwise supportive. If you wish more information on these devices and/or have other questions on male sexual dysfunction, contact the Association for Male Sexual Dysfunction, Suite 2-1 24 East 12th Street, New York, NY 10003, phone: 212-879-3131.

PENILE IMPLANTS

Penile prostheses or implants have been more widely used in the past to treat potency problems. However, they have fallen out of favor as a first-line treatment because of surgical complications and mechanical malfunction, as well as the widespread availability of drugs like Viagra. Currently prostheses are being provided only in complicated cases when Viagra and other treatments have not worked.

As of 1992, some 250,000 to 300,000 men in the United States had both inflatable and noninflatable prostheses of various types implanted, and in that same year the FDA began evaluating the safety of implants as medical devices. Such implants have been used to treat permanent organic erectile problems, especially those due to diabetes or vascular problems, and in a few instances, psychologically-based erectile difficulties that did not respond to psychotherapy.

These devices do not interfere with the pleasurable feelings of intercourse as long as a man's nerves of sensation in the genital area are in working order. Implants themselves do not guarantee a climax or increase sexual desire. Their main function is to produce a reliable erection. Those men who could have an orgasm before the surgery can generally do so afterward. The three main manufacturers of penile prostheses are American Medical Systems of Minnetonka, Minnesota, Mentor Corporation of Santa Barbara, California, and Dacomed of

Minneapolis, Minnesota. They will provide information about their products in response to letters and calls.

In order to reach a decision about the desirability of a penile implant you should know that the following are not considered good candidates for penile prosthesis:

- Men with untreated acute and severe depression. The depression should be successfully treated first.
- Those with serious psychosis or brain disease.
- Men with severe personality disorders, including the chronically dissatisfied.
- Those with severe and complicated marital problems.
- Men whose impotence is not clearly organic.
- Men who have health conditions that contraindicate elective surgery.

It is more advisable to consider a penile implant when

- Oral medications like Viagra do not work.
- It is clear that erectile difficulties are primarily a chronic organic problem (caused, for example, by diabetes or vascular disease or by problems associated with rectal or prostate surgery, pelvic nerve injury, or spinal cord injury).

- External devices do not work, and penile injections are not an option, or have failed.
- Sexual desire is strong and both you and your partner greatly value intercourse.
- You engage in sexual activity with your partner even in the absence of actual intercourse.
- The presence of erectile dysfunction per se is having a destructive effect on your relationship.
- As a couple you have a realistic understanding of what may be achieved, and both of you approve of the surgery. It is ideal if both you and your partner are involved in pre- and postsurgical consultation. Moreover, sex counseling in addition to the surgery is essential, since couples often need explicit instructions on how best to use a prosthesis.

What are the risks you encounter from such implants as these? There is always danger of infection at the time of insertion, as well as the possibility of mechanical malfunction. Current estimates of as high as 90 percent surgical success are likely exaggerated or, at the very least, based on unreliable data. In addition, satisfaction with a prosthesis may very well decline over time. The inflatable devices are reported to have a higher rate of failure and earlier prostheses often required another operation. Most such failures involve leaks from various parts of the apparatus, including saline leaks from the inflatable tubes.

Some believe that in general, implants are *not* considered to be lifetime devices, and will eventually need to be removed or replaced. Nonetheless, many urologists have a positive attitude about them, stating that current implants show vast improvements over earlier versions. The 1993 National Institutes of Health Consensus Conference on Impotence echoed this optimism, generally agreeing that implants represent an important treatment option for chronic potency problems. The U.S. Food and Drug Administration has begun requiring better monitoring of success rates on the part of doctors and better disclosure of problems by implant manufacturers.

REVASCULARIZATION

Arteriosclerosis and conditions such as peripheral vascular disease, sickle cell anemia, traumas or accidents to the penis and surrounding area, or simply an insufficient blood flow since birth can affect the circulation of blood to the penis. Revascularization, or surgery involving the shifting of blood vessels, is used to restore normal blood circulation to the penis. While this kind of surgery is still evolving, and results are currently disappointing, it shows some promise for the future. However, revascularization is almost never recommended for diabetic impotence. Some surgeons feel revascularization is not indicated in cases of advanced general arteriosclerosis. Others believe that arteriosclerosis often advances segmentally, and if it is more advanced in the penis than in other parts of the body, revascularization in that area may result in many more years of functioning. In one vascular condition, Leriche's syndrome, there is an intermittent reduction of the penile blood supply needed for erection. Aching, fatigue, weakness, cramping, numbness, discomfort in the thigh, pain in the calf, or limping may accompany this syndrome. Rest relieves many of the symptoms, and surgery can eliminate the limp and restore sexual potency.

SKIN PATCHES, TOPICAL OINTMENTS, AND SPRAYS

In 1992 research evidence began demonstrating that nitric oxide, a neurotransmitter, is involved in smooth muscle relaxation in the corpora cavernosa, thus making penile erection possible. This new understanding of the mechanism of tumescence has led to new treatment directions—and possibly the development of a removable patch of nitric oxide to be placed on the penis itself in order to keep it engorged and erect.

Skin patches, ointments, and sprays have not been very successful thus far but research is ongoing since topical application would be less physically invasive and less psychologically upsetting than injections, surgery, and the like. One product, Topiglan, a rub-on gel containing alprostadil, is currently in advanced clinical trials. It works by dilating blood vessels, thus causing erections.

QUESTIONABLE AND OFTEN DANGEROUS TREATMENTS FOR ERECTILE DYSFUNCTION

Because erectile dysfunction is such a widespread concern, a host of questionable treatments have evolved. Folklore is full of reputed "remedies." Doctors have been known to prescribe oysters, greens, and massive amounts of vitamins B_{12} and E. There are also "youth doctors" and nonmedical entrepreneurs who produce and sell countless substances and gadgets advertised to rejuvenate sexual potency. Older people are often the targets of fraudulent consumer schemes and devices that promise to "make you look younger" and "guarantee" to prevent or cure impotence. The U.S. Postal Service, which brings action against those engaged in obtaining money or property through the mail by means of false representations, provided us with a representative list of worthless nostrums and alleged aphrodisiacs. Among the popular names are "Mexican Spanish Fly in Liquid Form," "Instant Love Potion," "Sex Stimulant for Women," "Mad Dog Weed," "Magic Lure," "Super

Nature Tablets," "European Love Drops," "Linga Pendulum Penis Enlarger and Strengthener," "Big Ox," made of vitamins and minerals, an "herbal Viagra," rhino horn, and VBE-21, advertised as the "Doctor's Pill for Loss of Sex Drive." On pages 141–142, we list by popular and scientific names a variety of alleged aphrodisiacs. *Watch out for them.* If they seem to work, it is only through the power of suggestion, and any "cure" is likely to be temporary. Some are extremely dangerous. Spanish fly, for example, will not improve erections, yet some men continue to hope that it will work. An older man wrote us: "I wish you could tell me where I can get a small amount of Spanish fly. I will be careful with it as I am seventy-one and wouldn't want anything to go wrong." Our reply was to let him know that Spanish fly was not effective in improving erections and could possibly lead to death! Even small doses may produce kidney failure and shock within twenty-four hours. As for "herbal Viagra," some scientists say that it, along with various other dietary supplements, contains bovine or other animals' organs, tissues, and extracts that are not covered by regulation to protect consumers from animal products that might harbor "mad cow" prions!

The Food and Drug Administration (FDA) began an attempt to ban the sale of all nonprescription aphrodisiacs in mid-1985. The ban does not, however, cover products such as ginseng that do not claim to be aphrodisiacs but nevertheless have that association in the public mind. Chinese ginseng, readily available in health food stores, is used in the belief that it preserves health, increases alertness, and improves endurance. Its aphrodisiac action has been interpreted (but not scientifically proven) as a consequence of improved health, which produces a return to normal sexual desire and functioning. Taken in moderation, ginseng has no known adverse side effects.

Dozens of Internet Web sites along with health food stores tout one herb or another as "natural" and "alternative" treatments for sexual dysfunction. Herbs such as avena sativa, saw palmetto, schisandra, damiana, Siberian ginseng, bilberry, and gingko biloba have all developed reputations as aphrodisiacs for one condition or another. Two new herb products—Venix and ArginMax—have recently appeared containing ginkgo and L-arginine as well as other ingredients. The effectiveness of herbal remedies has not been demonstrated, nor have the side effects been reliably tested. Since they are sold outside of pharmacies—primarily in health food stores or over the Internet—their ingredients and potency are unregulated. Therefore, taking these products means taking a risk of unknown proportions.

Of all the aphrodisiacs, yohimbine is closest to living up to its reputation, now centuries old, as an effective drug for erectile dysfunction. The FDA has approved yohimbine for erectile treatment purposes. However, numerous researchers (including the German Commission E—the internationally recognized authority on herbs) still doubt its effectiveness and safety. Further studies are underway. Yohimbine is an extract from the bark of the West African yohimbe tree and is now available in the prescription drugs Yocon, Ahprodyne, Erex, Yohimex, and Yovitel. It is sold without prescription in health-food stores in many forms and under many names, including Super Man and Hot Stuff, but concentrations vary widely. Only the prescription drugs contain reliable amounts of yohimbine. As an alpha blocker, yohimbine induces dilation of certain blood vessels, increasing blood flow to the penis. Thus far it has been found to be modestly useful for this purpose, if given in high-enough dosages. But reports indicate that it may trigger panic attacks in men who are severely anxious. Its other possible side effects include sweating, headaches, nausea, mild tremors, heart palpitation, anxiety, mild blood pressure changes, and increased urinary output.

SOME FALSE APHRODISIACS

Alcohol (especially wines)

Cantharidin (tincture of *Cantharis vesicatoria* or "Spanish fly")

Capsicum (extract of *Capsicum frutescens*, which is cayenne pepper from South America)

Cimicifugin (resin from *Cimicifuga racemosa*, or black snakeroot)

Cubeb (Oleoresin from *Piper cubeba*, from Java)

Damiana (from leaves of *Turnera diffusa*, found in Mexico)

Ergot (Alkaloids from *Claviceps purpurea*)

Marijuana *(Cannabis sativa)*

Nux vomica (extract from seeds of *Strychnos nux-vomica*)

Sanguinaria (Extract from *Sanguinaria canadensis*, or bloodroot)

Vitamin E (d-alpha-tocopherol)

SOURCES OF INFORMATION ON ERECTILE DYSFUNCTION

Recently the diagnosis and treatment of erectile dysfunction has received unprecedented attention in the media and the medical community. There has been a rapid increase in the number of information and counseling centers set up throughout the country. Many of these centers and self-help groups have been formed by men with erectile problems and their partners, so that individuals and couples can receive medical and psychological support from both health professionals and people like themselves who have experienced the condition. The atmosphere at these self-help meetings is structured to be open, honest, and emotionally supportive. Read on for specific sources of information or counseling.

Impotence World Association (IWA), 119 S. Ruth St., Maryville, TN, 37803, and its American division, the *Impotence Institute of America (IIA)*, P.O. Box 410, Bowie, MD, 220-718-0410, Phone: 800-669-1605. This is the nation's only nonprofit independent health association exclusively dedicated to impotence education. For counseling and support, individuals and couples can contact Impotents Anonymous (IA), for men with erectile dysfunction, or I-ANON, for their partners. Founded in 1983, this nonprofit organization has numerous chapters throughout the United States and provides anonymous counseling and support. The organization also has audio- and videotapes on impotence, and offers a list of health-care professionals in your area who specialize in erectile problems. A free brochure, *Answers to the Most Often-Asked Questions About Impotence*, is available by calling 1-800-669-1603.

The Association for Male Sexual Dysfunction, E. Douglas Whitehead, M.D., 24 East 12th Street, Suite 2-1, New York, NY 10003, Phone: 212-879-3131, is a multispecialty group that offers evaluation, diagnosis, and treatment of male sexual dysfunctions. The specialties covered include urology, sex therapy, and psychiatry.

Impotence Information Center, P.O. Box 9, Minneapolis, MN 55440, Phone: 1-800-843-4315, is run by a maker of penile prostheses. A free booklet, *Impotence: Finding a Treatment Solution,* is available.

American Association of Sex Educators, Counselors, and Therapists (AASECT), P.O. Box 238, Mount Vernon, IA, 52314-0238, Phone: 319-895-8407, provides a list of its members in your state if you send a business-size self-addressed stamped envelope.

The Sexual Function Health Council of the American Foundation for Urologic Disease, Inc., 1128 North Charles Street, Baltimore, MD 21201, Phone: 800-242-2383, provides information and will answer questions on Peyronie's disease, prostate disease, erectile dysfunction, incontinence, and other urological disorders.

CHAPTER 6

❦

THE EFFECTS OF DRUGS (INCLUDING ALCOHOL) AND SURGERY ON YOUR SEXUALITY

DRUGS

Drugs—prescription or otherwise—can and do cause serious sexual problems for both men and women and are probably the number-one cause of sexual problems in men. Their impact on sexuality may be major or subtle. Doctors often fail to consider the sexual consequences of drugs they prescribe, and those who take them are often unaware that their medications may influence their sexual desire and/or functioning.

If you are having sexual problems, then it would be wise to consider whether the drugs you are using are having a negative impact on your sexuality. A study reported in 1983 in *The Journal of the American Medical Association* found that *25 percent* of sexual problems in men were either caused or complicated by medications. Less is known about the effects of drugs on female sexuality but the assumption is that those drugs that affect men will affect women as well. Some drugs interfere with the autonomic nervous system, which is involved in normal sexual response, while others affect mood and alertness or change the levels or action of sex hormones. Read on for more detailed information.

PRESCRIPTION DRUGS

Antianxiety medications, antidepressants, and certain antihypertensives (agents for controlling high blood pressure) have all been implicated in impaired erection in men. Their effects on women are less understood, largely because in the past, women were often not included in drug trials.

Antianxiety Medications (Tranquilizers)

Strong tranquilizers such as Mellaril (thioridazine) and other phenothiazines may cause failure to obtain an erection or to ejaculate even when the capacity for erection remains. Any tranquilizing drug—even mild ones such as Xanax and Valium—can also act as a depressant on both male and female sexual feelings.

Antidepressants

Reports indicate that 45 to 60 percent of those who take antidepressants, especially the selective serotonin reuptake inhibitors (SSRIs), experience an inability in reaching orgasm, or a delay or reduction in orgasm. Men often have erectile problems. Both men and women may also experience less sexual desire. The FDA states that the problem is much greater than first reported by drug companies. (Many drug package warnings put the figure of those affected at 2 to 4 percent—the FDA is now requiring that such figures be revised upward.) Adverse sexual side effects have been reported with many commonly used antidepressants, including Prozac, Zoloft, Paxil, Luvox, Tofranil, Nardil, Desyrel, and Effexor. Drugs like Remeron, Serzone, and possibly Celexa reportedly show less negative effect. Wellbutrin, the fourth–largest selling antidepressant, has also been found to cause fewer problems.

Physicians list several options to attempt to lessen sexual problems:

- Reduce the antidepressant dosage. (However, this may cause a relapse in the depression symptoms if the dosage goes too low.) Remember also that older people in general require lower dosages of most medications than younger people because of slower metabolism.
- Change the antidepressant. Some have more

sexual side effects than others and different people may respond differently to each medication. Serzone and Wellbutrin are thought to have less negative impact on sexuality.

• Take a "drug holiday" in which you discontinue medication briefly, usually for a weekend. Reportedly one may experience improvements with Zoloft and Paxil, for example, but not with Prozac. The reasons for this variation are still unknown. In addition, patients may experience troublesome withdrawal symptoms with brief "holidays."

• Use another medication as an antidote. For example, Wellbutrin has been given to good effect along with a person's regular antidepressant to help counteract sexual effects. The downside is that Wellbutrin may have its own side effects, including agitation. Some physicians have also tried adding BuSpar (an anti-anxiety drug), Ritalin (the attention deficit drug), yohimbine (for impotence), and ginkgo biloba, although there is little research to support such use. Psychostimulants, such as dextroamphetamine and methylphenidate (and surprisingly, even caffeine) are also being used with some reports of success. Patients are instructed to hold off on their dose of antidepressant one day before a sexual encounter. Then, an hour prior to sex, they take the psychostimulant. The antidepressant can be resumed thereafter.

There is a danger that both men and women will stop taking antidepressant medicine altogether because it interferes with sex. However, one must weigh the impact of the sexual side effects against the need for the antidepressant and act accordingly. Two more points to remember: First, not everyone necessarily experiences the side effects, and second, because depression itself can cause loss of sexual desire, the successful treatment of depression in and of itself may restore sexual desire and response.

Several studies on men and on very small samples of women have shown Viagra to be useful in counteracting the negative sexual effects of antidepressants. However, these studies are preliminary, especially for women, and larger clinical trials are needed.

Antihypertensives

Antihypertensive medications are the most common cause of impaired erection. Blocking agents, one class of antihypertensive drugs, include methyldopa (Aldomet), which reduces the flow of blood into the pelvic area and so inhibits erection.

Thomas, sixty-two, had always believed himself to be in good health, and was surprised when his physician told him he had high blood pressure. The doctor recommended changes in his diet, as well as an exercise program. Thomas's blood pressure improved somewhat, but still ran about 130 over 95. The doctor thought it important that Thomas be on antihypertensive medication, and put him on methyldopa. Thomas's blood pressure was soon under control, but as a consequence of the drug, he was often unable to have an erection. He discussed this with his physician, and once an angiotensin-converting enzyme (ACE) inhibitor, a class of antihypertensive agents that appear to have fewer adverse effects on sexuality, was substituted for methyldopa, Thomas's erection problems disappeared. (Sometimes efforts to vary or lower the dosage of antihypertensive medications are not always so successful; however, in Thomas's case, things worked out well.)

Another drug used against hypertension, guanethidine (Ismelin), may inhibit ejaculation by blocking the nerves involved. Up to two-thirds of men taking this medication have reported problems. Guanethidine can also cause retrograde ejaculation. The antihypertensive reserpine can decrease sexual interest or, at times, induce erectile dysfunction. Even the diuretics given for high blood pressure can cause problems, as Bob, age sixty-eight, found out when he was placed on a diuretic for this very problem. When he was unable to have an erection, it never occurred to him that the diuretic might be responsible. He attributed his changing status to aging. Fortunately, his physician asked him if there were any side effects from the medication, specifically in terms of his erectile function. When the doctor learned of Bob's problem, he lowered the dosage of the medication and Bob soon reported returning to normal.

The antihypertensive drugs that are frequently implicated in impaired sexuality include those with peripheral and central actions of sympatholytic or beta-adrenergic blocking activity. Most importantly, calcium channel blockers, ACE inhibitors, and peripheral vasodilators *do not* cause significant sexual dysfunction.

If you develop sexual problems after taking antihypertensive medications, *don't* discontinue or decrease your medications without telling your doctor. Doing so would be very dangerous, as your medications could be preventing a stroke.

Your doctor may be able to help solve your sexual problems without endangering your health. Some alternatives are to switch antihypertensives, to use only a diuretic, and/or to reduce dosages when feasible. In fact, many physicians no longer prescribe medications for mild to moderate hypertension until their patients have first tried to bring their blood pressure under control by lowering salt intake and by exercise and weight reduction. When drugs *are* necessary, one study suggests that one of the most effective regimens—with the least likelihood of sexual impairment—is a combination of an oral diuretic, hydralazine, and propranolol (Inderal). However, propranolol, promoted at first for its lack of sexual side effects, has now been implicated as affecting sexuality, especially when higher dosages are used.

Other Drugs

What other drugs should you be concerned about? The corticosteroids taken for arthritis may produce at least temporary erectile difficulties. Analgesics (pain medications) may reduce sensitivity and, therefore, affect male sexual capacity. Cimetidine (Tagamet), used in the treatment of duodenal ulcers and one of the most widely sold medicines in the United States, can cause problems. One possible substitute for cimetidine that should not impair your sexuality is ranitidine (Zantac). Digoxin (Lanoxin) for antiarrhythmias, levodopa (Dopar and Larodopa) for Parkinsonism, and the antiseizure drugs carbamazepine (Atretol and Tegretol), phenytoin (Dilantin), and primidone (Myidone and Mysoline) can all cause sexual dysfunction. Danazol (Danocrine) for endometriosis and dichlorphenamide (Daranide) for glaucoma are also problematic, as are antipsychotic medications, including Thorazine, Mellaril, and lithium.

ALCOHOL

You should be aware that alcohol is also a drug. Pharmacologically it is a depressant rather than a stimulant, though in small amounts it may relax sexual inhibition in a pleasant manner. In larger amounts, however, it usually interferes with sexual performance, reducing potency in males and arousal and orgasmic ability in both sexes. At the very least, alcohol often produces drowsiness, which then interferes with sex. The excessive use of alcohol is a frequent and too-little-recognized factor in sexual problems, and often those who abuse alcohol fail to realize how much they are actually drinking.

Certainly, most people would never have realized that Mary, age sixty-five, had a drinking problem. Mary herself never suspected it. Over the years, especially since her husband's death, she had begun drinking more frequently. Rather than one or two drinks a day, she now regularly had at least three or four. Since her husband's death, various men had expressed interest in her, but Mary had lost all sexual desire. She considered this a kind of loyalty to her husband. During her annual visit to her doctor, he asked about her alcohol intake and began to suspect alcohol abuse. Mary denied having a problem. But one day she had a serious fall on the stairs that even she could see had been related to her drinking. Her doctor strongly recommended that she go to the Hazelton alcohol treatment center in Minnesota for treatment. She took his advice and some months later, was recovering and doing quite well. Moreover, she was surprised to find that her sexual feelings and desires had returned.

How does alcohol intake affect the members of both sexes? For men, even a few drinks before sex can impair sexual performance. Erections may be less firm and ejaculation more difficult. But though this effect is temporary and reversible in terms of physical capacity, it can frighten a man into believing he is impotent, and the fear itself may then prolong the difficulty.

Up to 80 percent of men who drink heavily are believed to suffer serious sexual side effects, including sexual dysfunction, sterility, or loss of sexual desire. Many of the effects of moderate to heavy drinking may be reversible if the drinking stops in time. However, heavy drinking over a long period irreversibly destroys testicular cells, leaving men with shrunken testicles. Both sexual drive and sexual capacity can be damaged. Hormone production is often affected, resulting in a decrease in the sperm count. Total sterility as well as erectile dysfunction result. Chronic heavy drinking can also produce liver and brain damage that leads to an excess production of female hormones and a feminized body appearance.

Women are affected by alcohol in many of the same ways as men. More than one drink before a sexual encounter can interfere with arousal and the ability to reach orgasm. Chronic heavy use of alcohol in the middle years can damage the ovaries, causing menstrual and ovulatory abnormalities and a decrease in estrogen production. This in turn may lead to early menopause and signs of premature aging. Atrophy of the breasts, uterus, and vaginal walls and lessened lubrication in the vagina are common.

One's tolerance for alcohol decreases with age (one cause is changing kidney excretory power), so that smaller and smaller amounts may begin to produce negative effects. It is wise to avoid drinking altogether for several hours before a sexual encounter, or at least to limit alcohol intake to one drink. If you choose to drink regularly, limit yourself to a maximum of one and a half ounces of hard liquor, one six-ounce glass of wine, or two eight-ounce glasses of beer in any twenty-four-hour period. Remember, too, that alcohol is very dangerous in combination with narcotic and nonnarcotic drugs such as sleeping pills, sedatives, painkillers, antihistamines, antidepressants, and tranquilizers, because it can pyramid their effects. So *if you are taking drugs, do not drink without first discussing it with your doctor.*

Total abstinence is the only viable treatment for alcoholism. The "moderation" approach does not work. Alcoholics Anonymous, counseling, and medications such as Atabuse remain the best treatment methods.

TOBACCO

Because of its nicotine content, tobacco is also a drug. It can be a factor in erectile difficulties, with some studies showing that smokers are 50 percent more likely than nonsmokers to have potency problems before the age of fifty. There is an old German saying about male erectile capacity: *"Rauchen macht schlump"*—"Smoking makes [it] dangle." A recent antismoking television message in the United States depicted a limp, drooping cigarette with the caption "Cigarettes: Still Think They're Sexy?" By 1998, cigarette packages in Thailand were required to carry the warning "Cigarette smoking causes sexual impotence"— probably the first example of a comprehensive preventive effort of this kind by any nation.

Toxic changes in the blood from nicotine affect sex hormones. There is some evidence that men who smoke have lower levels of testosterone and lower sperm counts. Nicotine also constricts blood vessels, in some cases enough to affect blood flow to the penis. Long-term smokers who also suffer from atherosclerosis or peripheral vascular disease have a much higher chance of erectile dysfunction than that caused by vascular disease alone. Studies suggest that smoking per se, regardless of number of years spent smoking or the number of cigarettes per day, has an immediate negative effect on potency. Therefore, any smoking behavior should be a consideration when a man is having erectile difficulties.

It is also suspected that smoking affects female sexual capacity, but this issue has received little specific research attention. It is known that tobacco use can be linked to an early menopause as well as heart disease, lung cancer, and a large number of other conditions. Smoking studies have also focused on the impact on women's physical appearance. Recent research by British dermatologists (reported in the medical journal *Lancet*) found that a gene activated by tobacco destroys collagen, leading to premature wrinkling of the skin.

NARCOTICS AND OTHER DRUGS

Regular users of opiates like morphine, heroin, and even methadone are often sexually impaired. Males who are addicted are usually impotent.

While cocaine initially heightens sexual sensation in both sexes as a result of euphoria, increased energy, and heightened self-confidence, with its habitual use individuals experience a lowered sense of self-esteem, together with insomnia, fatigue, anxiety, depression, and even paranoia, hallucinations, and seizures. Women become nonorgasmic and men impotent. A national telephone aid line—1-800-662-HELP—has been established by the American Council for Drug Education for those who want help in stopping cocaine use.

Marijuana can lead to decreased sexual interest and impotence as well as the drying out of the mucous membranes in the sex organs. Amphetamines can produce erectile dysfunction, delayed or no ejaculation in men, and inhibition of orgasms in women. Regular users of such barbiturates as sedatives and hypnotics (sleeping pills) may also be adversely affected sexually.

A rare but exceedingly destructive condition called priapism can occur in men who use certain drugs such as butyl (or isobutyl) nitrate, known also as poppers, to stimulate more frequent and longer-lasting erections. An antidepressant drug, trazodone (Desyrel), can also cause similar problems. Priapism is a persistent and often painful erection of the penis caused by blood becoming trapped in the corpora cavernosa—the chambers in the penis that fill with blood to create erections. The erection does not subside on its own, and emergency medical care is needed within twenty-four hours or less to avoid permanent damage to the penis and almost certain permanent impotence. Partial priapism—any unusual period of persistent erection that eventually goes away by itself—is a sign that something is wrong; seek medical advice and treatment.

AVOIDING PROBLEMS

Health-care professionals who prescribe or monitor the use of drugs should be thoroughly familiar with each drug's potential for adverse effects on sexuality. (See the section on drugs and sexuality in *The Merck Manual of Geriatrics* [Merck Research Laboratories, 2000].) It is important that doctors obtain their patients' sexual history before giving any drug that may affect sexuality. This allows comparisons to be made before and after drugs are taken. Physicians should review their patients' drug usage regularly, including their use of prescription and other over-the-counter drugs, alcohol, and tobacco. Plus, doctors should carefully explain the potential side effects of drugs to their patients.

Most drug-caused sexual impairment is reversible if the responsible drug is reduced, removed, or replaced by another. (Impairment due to chronic alcoholism and possibly heavy and chronic marijuana use may *not* be reversible.) In cases of serious illness, sexuality may have to be partially—or even totally—sacrificed for a period of time in order to obtain the beneficial effects of drugs that are essential to treatment. But in many cases, alternative drugs, lower dosages, or other treatment altogether can be given. For example, an antihypertensive drug that may adversely affect one person's sexuality will not affect another's. Weigh the possible sexual side effects of a drug against the risks of a disease; your—the patient's—preference should be a crucial factor in the resulting decision.

SURGERY

It is certainly not surprising that most people are apprehensive about any and all surgery on their sex organs. In addition to the usual risks involved in any surgical procedure, they dread possible sexual consequences. Many women mistakenly believe removal of the womb (hysterectomy) or of a breast (mastectomy) makes them "less of a woman." And men worry that prostate surgery means the end of a sex life altogether. It is reassuring to know that the medical evidence does not support many of these fears, as long as the surgeons are skilled, knowledgeable about the possible problems, and sensitive to their patients' interest in preserving sexual functioning.

HYSTERECTOMY

A hysterectomy is the removal of the womb or uterus. In addition, the ovaries and Fallopian tubes may also be removed (this is called bilateral salping-oophorectomy). It is estimated that more than half of all women will have had a hysterectomy by age sixty-five, making this the most common major operation performed in the United States on women unrelated to pregnancy. However, the rate has dropped considerably since the 1970s as evidence accumulated showing that a proportion of these operations—such as those performed to remove the ovaries and uterus as a preventative against future cancers in these organs—are unnecessary. The slim risk of contracting cancer must be weighed against the many benefits of avoiding such surgeries. In fact, hysterectomy is now described as "last-resort" surgery for a number of conditions that previously would have warranted this measure. If you are considering a hysterectomy, we strongly suggest that you receive a second, or even a third, opinion. Hysterectomy Educational Resources and Services (HERS) offers free phone counseling and support to women and their families faced with the question of surgery. For a free packet of information about hysterectomy and HERS services, write 422 Bryn Mawr Avenue, Bala Cynwyd, PA 19004, Phone: 610-667-7757. HERS also distributes a quarterly newsletter. The National Women's Health Network, 514 10th Street N.W., Suite 400, Washington, DC, 20004, Phone:

202-628-7814, also provides an information packet on hysterectomy for a small fee.

Many hysterectomies are done because of the presence of benign (noncancerous) tumors called fibroids, which are not troublesome so long as they remain small but may require surgery if they enlarge, cause bleeding, or involve other organs. Endometriosis, prolapse of the uterus ("fallen uterus"); cancer of the cervix, the endometrium (lining of the uterus), or related organs; and severe, uncontrollable infection or bleeding are other legitimate reasons for a hysterectomy.

It is often said there is no medical evidence that the careful removal of the uterus causes impairment of sexual sensations. Yet some women greatly depend on sensations from the cervix and womb to achieve orgasm through deep penile penetration; after hysterectomy they must learn other methods of arousal, such as more focus on clitoral response. The rhythmic contractions of the uterus during orgasm are gone, of course, as a result of a hysterectomy. During the surgical repair, surgeons should be careful to avoid shortening the vagina, which can lead to problems with intercourse. Correct positioning of the wound repair in the back of the vagina is also important. If intercourse is resumed too early after hysterectomy, there can be pain due to incomplete healing in the vagina. Most physicians recommend waiting six to eight weeks before sexual activity is begun again.

Many surgeons and women themselves warn that a period of emotional instability commonly begins about the third or fourth day after a hysterectomy and lasts two to five or ten days or longer. Depression, sleep disturbances, fatigue, listlessness, weight gain, loss of appetite, weeping, and irritability may occur—they are physical and/or emotional responses to the surgery. If symptoms are severe or long lasting, they may require psychotherapeutic, hormonal, or other interventions. Most women regain their equilibrium naturally, although many claim that it takes six months or longer to fully recover physically, especially if the ovaries have been removed.

Removal of all or parts of a woman's childbearing apparatus, powerful symbols of womanhood, often does have significant psychological effects. If the woman sees the surgery as symbolic "castration," she needs to resolve this, either on her own or with outside help. She must understand that removal of the sexual organs need not eradicate sexuality, cause her to feel unattractive, or diminish her womanliness. Short-term preoperative and postoperative counseling, ideally with her partner present, can do much to allay a woman's fears and misapprehensions. Group discussions with other women who have had hysterectomies can be especially helpful; women's health centers or hospital social workers may be able to arrange this.

Hysterectomies *can* have positive effects on sexuality, particularly if they are done to relieve painful or debilitating conditions like infection, urinary incontinence, heavy bleeding, or endometriosis. A return to pain-free good health can be a potent aphrodisiac! A recent two-year posthysterectomy study of over one thousand women by four women faculty members at the University of Maryland Medical School (reported in *The Journal of the American Medical Association*) found that sexual relations increased after hysterectomy, along with a greater desire for sex, an increased incidence of orgasm, and—significantly—a drastic decrease in pain during intercourse.

MASTECTOMY

While most breast lumps (80 to 90 percent) are found to be benign upon biopsy, unfortunately the likelihood of breast cancer increases with age. A lumpectomy or a full or partial breast removal or mastectomy, is performed when a lump in the breast is found to be malignant (cancerous).

In spite of current controversy over whether breast cancer begins in the breast or is a systemic disease beginning elsewhere, most physicians emphasize the early detection of lumps as a major means of combating the disease. In addition to routine examination by your physician and the use of newer techniques to help him or her in diagnosis (for example, yearly mammography by low-voltage X rays), you should definitely undertake regular monthly self-examinations. For information on breast cancer, call the Cancer Information Service at the National Cancer Institute, Bethesda, MD 20003, 1-800-422-6237.

There are different kinds of mastectomy, ranging from removal of only the lump(s) and some adjacent tissue to the removal of the entire breast, the surrounding lymph glands, and chest muscles. These operations have understandable psychological implications for many women, because they not only change the outward appearance of the body but also visibly alter a specific symbol of sexuality. Periodic depression, with its subsequent consequences for one's sex life, is common and expected during the first year or two after a mastectomy. Aesthetic reactions to breast removal can be more difficult than with a hysterectomy, which leaves no obvious signs beyond an abdominal scar.

Although there is no known physiological change in sexual capacity after mastectomy, women may temporarily lose their sexual desire out of embarrassment, inability to accept the loss of the breast, and fear that they have become less attractive to their sexual partners. They are also afraid the absence of the breast will be noticeable in public. Some women choose breast reconstruction, using either silicone or saline implants or tissue from elsewhere in the body. However, in 1992 the FDA ordered sharp reductions in the use of silicone-gel breast implants until extensive studies of their safety could be carried out. Saline implants are also under study. (For up-to-date information on implants, call the

National Cancer Institute's Information Service at 1-800-422-6237.) To immediately relieve anxiety about their public appearance, women can choose to wear a properly fitting prosthetic bra. However, reactions to breast loss by the women themselves and their partners are not always so easily resolved.

One useful technique is to talk frankly with other women who have already experienced a breast loss. Some physicians and hospitals arrange for such volunteers to counsel women prior to and following surgery. The Reach to Recovery program of the American Cancer Society, begun by Terese Lazar in 1952, is a rehabilitation program for women who have had breast surgery. (A helpful free booklet, *Reach to Recovery*, is available from local units of the American Cancer Society.) The program is designed to help with physical, psychological, and cosmetic concerns, and utilizes a carefully selected and trained corps of volunteers who have adjusted successfully to their own surgery. Other forms of individual and group support can be immensely relieving as well.

Men, too, need a period of adjustment to work out their feelings about breast surgery in their partners. In some cities, Reach to Recovery uses male volunteers to help men adjust to their wives' mastectomies, while The Cancer Care Foundation and numbers of other organizations have support groups for cancer patients' "significant others." In strong relationships, time and affection often take care of any disturbed feelings following the removal of a breast.

When Hannah, age sixty, received a phone call from her physician telling her that her mammogram looked suspicious, she hurried in to be examined. A small lump was found. She and her husband were hoping, of course, that it would be benign at biopsy. Unfortunately, that was not the case; she had cancer. After exploring various possibilities, Hannah had a mastectomy of her left breast. She was given a good chance of recovery because the cancer had been found early. But Hannah was anxious about her appearance. At first she would not let her husband see or touch her scar; however, he wisely insisted. Now she says, "I had more trouble dealing with it than my husband." Both report that they have become comfortable and feel even more tender toward one another than before the operation.

However, severe and prolonged emotional upset may require professional psychotherapy. Do not avoid seeking aid in such cases; the odds are that it will help greatly, whether the problem lies with you or with your mate.

To speed up the resumption of a normal sex life after a mastectomy, you should practice the following:

- Involve your partner in all aspects of the discussions around a mastectomy.
- Have your partner see the surgical repair as early as possible after surgery, so the process of adjustment can begin.
- Resume sexual activity as soon as possible.

- Find comfortable sexual positions. For the first weeks and perhaps months, your surgical repair will be sensitive. A preferred sexual position is to have your partner on top, supporting his upper body with his arms. This leaves you in a relaxed position on your back, with no stress on your chest area.
- Decide together whether you want to wear a prosthesis (a padded bra or a bodylike form that fits in a bra) during sexual contact or whether you, as a couple, can be comfortable without it. Many couples eventually eliminate the need for the cover-up.
- Share feelings openly and support each other emotionally. Both of you are likely to have periods of depression and anxiety due to the fear of death that cancer brings and to the loss of a valued body part. Those who can share such feelings may not need further counseling after the initial adjustment period.

Methods of breast cancer treatment remain highly controversial. Some years ago most surgeons routinely performed what is called the Halsted radical mastectomy. It involved removing the entire breast, underlying muscles, and the nearby lymph nodes, thereby leaving a woman with a sunken chest wall and impaired mobility of the arm. When it was discovered that surgeons in countries such as Canada and England were removing much less breast tissue and getting nearly identical survival rates, American surgeons began changing their approach. Many now perform either a modified radical mastectomy, which removes less muscle and fewer lymph nodes, or lumpectomies, which remove only the lump itself. These surgeries have been found to be equally as effective as the more radical procedures. Radiation and chemotherapy (described next) may be used as well.

Drug therapies, also called adjuvant therapy, are the additional treatment that cancer specialists use, along with the surgery, to improve survival chances. Tamoxifen, an artificial hormone that blocks estrogen, is widely used. Advances in chemotherapy—drugs that attack cancer cells—are promising.

VAGINAL RECONSTRUCTION

Women who have had a number of children, difficult childbirths, or tears in the opening of the vagina at the time of childbirth may have an excessively enlarged vagina. Anterior and posterior plastic repair, a surgical procedure, may reconstruct the vagina effectively and make sex more pleasurable. This is a delicate operation and requires an especially skilled surgeon who is also sensitive to the woman's needs. We recommend a second medical opinion on the advisability of this surgery.

PROSTATECTOMY

Prostatectomy involves surgical removal of part or all of the prostate, a gland located at the base of the urethra. As men grow older, up to half of them experience significant enlargement of the prostate. This usually begins after age forty or fifty, and almost all men over fifty have some degree of enlargement. Fifty to 75 percent have noticeable symptoms and at least half eventually require surgery. By the time men reach the age of eighty prostate enlargement is almost universal, although in a few cases the prostate gland atrophies with extreme age. No one knows yet why the prostate undergoes growth in midlife after a period of dormancy following adolescence. There is evidence that African American men develop prostate enlargement an average of five years earlier than white men. There also appear to be lower rates of enlargement among non-American Asian men compared to American Asian men. Diet may be a factor, especially large amounts of fat. Some physicians believe a zinc deficiency may be involved, but there is no solid evidence for this. Zinc taken in small doses will do no harm, but it is not a medically proved treatment or preventive for prostate problems.

When the enlargement is noncancerous, as is usually the case, it is called benign prostatic hyperplasia (too many cells), or BPH. BPH starts very gradually and may exist for years with no symptoms. In fact, many men remain symptomless throughout their lives except for the enlargement.

The size of the enlarged prostate gland is less significant than the amount of obstruction it produces at the neck of the bladder. Since the prostate gland is so close to the bladder and urethra, the enlargement can produce a number of problems with urination. Men may find themselves with some or all of the following symptoms: An enlarged prostate may increase the need and urgency to urinate or to get up to void during the night. There may be a delay in starting the stream of urine, a slowness or weakness in the stream, or even a total inability to urinate. Occasionally, small amounts of blood are present in the urine and during ejaculation. (Bleeding should *always* be medically evaluated, since it could also be a symptom of cancer.) The dribbling of urine after urination is common and requires the use of paper tissues for a few minutes to catch the drops of urine. Since enlargement of the gland may lead to retention and stagnation of urine, there can also be bacterial infection. In severe and untreated cases, damage is done to the kidneys. Surgery may be necessary when a urinary shutdown occurs.

The causes of noncancerous prostatic difficulties are unknown but may be connected to a genetic predisposition, to changes in endocrine levels, and/or to aging processes. Previous theories about changes in hormone levels seem to have been disproved at Johns Hopkins Medical School and elsewhere. A curious aspect of BPH is that it has been found in aging men and aging dogs, but in no other species. We also should mention that there is no foundation to the folklore that prostate trouble is related to "excessive" sexual activity. Indeed, evidence suggests that an active and regular sex life preserves healthy prostate functioning, while a pattern of irregular ejaculations may lead to such problems as inflammation.

Advances in the medical (including hormonal) treatment of BPH also seem promising. For example, Hytrin, a brand of terazosin, relieves pressure on the urethra almost immediately and mitigates symptoms in about two-thirds of prostate patients by its effects on the muscles. It does have some untoward side effects, such as dizziness and fatigue, and has been reported to cause ED in some patients.

The drug Proscar shrinks the prostate somewhat and appears to be free of major side effects. With Proscar, it takes about three months before the prostate shrinks enough to relieve symptoms. The drug specifically blocks 5-alpha reductase, the enzyme that converts testosterone to dihydrotestosterone, the hormone associated with the growth of the prostate gland. Of those treated with Proscar, 3.7 percent became impotent, whereas 1.6 percent of those on a placebo reported impotence. A 3.3 percentage of the Proscar subjects also reported decreased sexual desire. Impotence and lack of desire are dose dependent and prove to be reversible once the patient stops taking the drug.

A new treatment for BPH that uses a laser is

currently being tested. The YAG laser is an intense light beam that can be used under local anesthesia to destroy the excess prostate tissue in benign prostatic enlargement. The tissue is then voided with the urine. The advantage of the laser is that it avoids other surgical procedures and allows the extra tissue to be painlessly eliminated. This is still in its experimental stages, however, and is not yet available for the general public. There is also the balloon treatment, in which a tiny balloon is run through a catheter to the prostate gland and inflated with high pressure for several minutes, to open up the urethra. Its side effects are few, and for some, this treatment seems effective. Yet, at present, a prostatectomy to treat the BPH remains the treatment of choice, with 400,000 prostatectomies being performed each year. (Twenty percent of those who undergo this surgery must undergo a second operation within ten years.) Some doctors now recommend surgery at an early point in the course of symptoms to avoid unnecessary complications and dire emergencies; this is a decision best made jointly by you and your doctor. There are three types of prostatectomies, all of which require anesthesia:

Transurethral resection, or TUR, is the most common, least traumatic, and safest surgical procedure because it requires no outside incision. A thin, hollow, fiber-optic tube is inserted in the penis, an electric loop is maneuvered through the tube, and the prostate gland is removed. One disadvantage of this technique is that the tissue sometimes grows back. TUR is recommended chiefly when the prostate is not too enlarged, and for men over seventy.

Suprapubic or retropubic surgery (named for the site of the incision, above or behind the pubic bone) is performed when the gland is very large. The tissue is removed through an incision made in the abdomen.

Perineal surgery is used by some surgeons for men with substantial prostate enlargement who are in poor physical condition. There is very little postoperative bleeding or pain with this procedure. An even more radical perineal procedure is used in the surgical treatment of cancer of the gland. These procedures can be performed with a high degree of safety even on a very old man. An incision is made in the perineum between the scrotum and the anus, and most or all of the prostate is removed. Whether surgery is more effective than radiotherapy for operable prostate cancer is unknown. Radiotherapy, however, results in impotence in 30 to 60 percent of men, compared to the nearly 100 percent impotence perineal surgery causes.

Potency is rarely affected by the TUR and suprapubic procedures, and some men actually experience increased potency because their prostatic problems have been eliminated. It is generally agreed that 80 percent of men return to their presurgery sexual functioning, 10 percent actually have improved sexual functioning, while 10 percent have some or even total loss of the ability to achieve an erection. (Fifteen percent of those

who have had TUR experience some urinary incontinence.) The perineal approach—especially the radical
procedure—has been the chief physical cause of impotence following prostatic surgery because it requires
critical nerves to be cut. Perineal surgery also may affect
the ability to urinate by causing strictures to form in the
urethra. Dilation of the urethra is then required.

Prior to surgery, prostate problems usually do not
interfere with sexual functioning unless pain is present.
Some men may experience a slight decrease in the force
of their ejaculation, but others may have benign prostate
problems for years with no change in sexual functioning. After a prostatectomy, particularly for those operations done for BPH as we have noted, most men resume
normal sexual activity. Healing time runs at least six
weeks, and most men wait four to six weeks before resuming sexual activity. The only sexual change after
most types of surgery is that in many cases semen is no
longer ejaculated through the penis but instead is
pushed backward into the bladder (retrograde ejaculation), where it is voided with the urine. This so-called
dry ejaculation happens because a space has been left
where the enlarged prostate had been, and fluid travels
the path of least resistance to the bladder. Although men
in this situation can no longer father children, the large
majority have erections as before, with no diminishment
of sexual pleasure. (However, if couples wish, sperm can
be successfully extracted from the urine and deposited
in the younger female partner's vagina for fertilization

purposes.) It is important not to depend on retrograde ejaculation for birth control, however, since some semen may still pass down through the penis. In addition, normal ejaculation may very well return following some regrowth of the prostate; in such instances, fertility may be restored. (A certain amount of regrowth can occur without causing difficulties or requiring surgery.)

By far the greatest cause of erectile difficulties occurring with prostatectomies is *psychological*. Unfortunately, family doctors and urologists do not always provide adequate information about what to expect after surgery, so that a man falsely assumes sexual impairment. This assumption, with its consequent fear, is based on the tendency to associate the prostate gland with the penis, since the two are in physical proximity.

And beware of the many quack remedies that promise treatment without surgery. Various kinds of massage, foods, and other "cures," often at exorbitant prices, are offered to men seeking a quick cure for a sometimes serious condition. Avoid them and rely instead on your physician's advice.

Prostate Cancer

Cancer of the prostate, a much more serious disorder than BPH, occurs largely in men over sixty. Its cause is still unknown. It does not appear that men with BPH have higher rates of prostate cancer than those without BPH. Most such cancers are not detected until men are in their seventies. *Cancer of the prostate is the second leading cause of cancer deaths in men,* killing 32,000 annually. Each year 180,000 men are diagnosed with prostate cancer. Studies reveal that almost half of all men under age seventy have at least microscopic prostate tumors and 80 percent to 90 percent have such signs by age eighty and older, although most older men die of other conditions first. The probability of developing prostate cancer in one's lifetime is about 8 percent for American men. A family history of prostate cancer doubles the risk, especially if more than one relative had the disease, and if it had been acquired at a relatively young age (as in the fifties). A high-fat diet appears to be a risk factor. African American men tend to develop a more lethal prostate cancer, for reasons yet unclear.

Early detection is critical. The five-year survival rate is 100 percent for men whose cancer at the time of diagnosis is confined to the prostate. However, the rate decreases to 30 percent survival the first five years for those whose cancer has spread to other parts of the body.

When detected early, many cases can be successfully treated with surgery and/or radiation (delivered externally or implanted as "seeds") or other treatments. Most men choose surgery; however, a high percentage of men (60 percent or more) have some degree of erectile dysfunction afterward. While all methods are effective against the cancer, surgery may be more curative, especially in the younger patient. About 25 percent of men choosing surgery will also require radiation, because of evidence that the cancer has spread. Originally radiation as the first line of defense was thought to be more protective of potency; however, it has now been found that a significant number of men who undergo this treatment—30 to 60 percent—do experience permanent impotence. Both surgery and radiation may also result in urinary incontinence.

Cryosurgery is another option. This procedure involves freezing the cancerous tissue by pumping cold gas into probes that have been inserted into the prostate.

Chemotherapy (cis-platin or vincristine) and hormone therapy are also commonly used in the treatment of prostatic cancer. During the course of chemotherapy, problems with erections and desire may emerge, but they do disappear after the therapy has stopped. Hormone therapy involves either bilateral orchiectomy (removal of both testicles) or hormones (e.g., Lupron, a hormone that turns off the pituitary gland and thereby reduces testosterone), or a combination of both. The intent of hormone therapy is to eliminate the testosterone that feeds this cancer. Side effects can include a decrease in sexual desire and difficulties in erection. Oral sildenafil (Viagra), penile injections, or vacuum devices can counteract the impotence (see pages 118–136), but testosterone treatments should not be given.

A physical exam at least once a year after age forty, including a digital (finger) rectal examination (DRE) and a complete urinalysis, greatly enhances the chance of early detection. The PSA blood test performed at the

time of the DRE is still controversial in terms of diagnostic usefulness. Some of the cancers detected by PSA
might not pose a threat if untreated. Some say if a man
has a life expectancy of ten years or less, he should not
have a PSA test. A normal PSA is below four, a high
is above ten. Inflamed or enlarged prostates can cause
elevated readings. Proscar, Propecia, and the herb
saw palmetto lower PSA. BPH can raise the PSA. False
PSA positives are common and can lead to unnecessary
biopsies.

A prostate biopsy involves a biopsy gun that shoots
a needle into the prostate to remove tissue in a fraction
of a second. A Gleason grade (one to ten) scores the
character of cancer cells from low to high in terms of
their aggressiveness. The patient feels distinct pain in the
prostate during the biopsy.

Cancer of the prostate is relatively slow growing
and may go through dormant periods. Indeed "watchful
waiting" is the treatment of choice for most men after
age seventy-five, especially if they have low prostate specific antigen (PSA) and low Gleason grade.

In 1982, a nerve-sparing operation (a modified
radical retropubic prostatectomy), designed to protect
the nerve centers damaged by the usual cancer surgery,
was developed at Johns Hopkins by Dr. Patrick C. Walsh
(see Walsh's book, *The Prostate: A Guide for Men and the
Women Who Love Them*, Warner Books, 1997). This
nerve-sparing surgery has been incorporated into a
prostate cancer operation called radical perineal prostec-

tomy, which is rapidly gaining favor. Many urologists now offer such surgery, which preserves potency in 70 percent or more of those who successfully undergo the operation. There is, however, considerable anatomical variation and also little margin for error, making this one of the most difficult surgeries to perform correctly. A new device, known as CaverMap, is being used by some surgeons to refine their surgical technique—however, not all agree on its usefulness.

Male Incontinence

Today there are many treatment options to help with urinary incontinence whether or not there has been surgery performed for an enlarged prostate or to treat cancer of the prostate. The implantation of a urinary prosthesis can control the flow of urine for approximately 90 percent of those men who undergo insertions of a urinary sphincter. For more information on bladder control problems, including incontinence, contact The National Association for Continence, P.O. Box 8310, Spartanburg, SC 29305-8310, Phone: 1-800-252-3337.

ORCHIECTOMY

This surgery, which is removal of the testes, may help control cancer of the prostate. The psychological impact of this castration can be devastating. Emotional preparation before and counseling following the surgery are absolutely indispensable. The placement of artificial testes (made of plastic or tantalum) may be advisable for both cosmetic and emotional reasons. Impotence does not always follow removal of the testes; some 10 percent of men having this surgery do continue to have normal erections. Usually ejaculations no longer occur, although there may be a little prostate fluid.

COLOSTOMY AND ILEOSTOMY

When part of the bowel must be removed for lifesaving purposes, the anus is generally closed and an artificial opening in the abdomen created. The surgery may be in the colon (colostomy) or in the ileum (an ileostomy). Needless to say, the patient has many sensitive adjustments to make after such surgery. A bag attached to the opening fills with feces and must be emptied, although many colostomy patients develop enough bowel predictability to simply wear a gauze pad. There are possible embarrassing bowel sounds as well as odors, although much of this can be adequately controlled. Those who undergo ostomies have to work their way through their own feelings, as well as their perceptions of other people's attitudes. And the most complicated issue of all can be working out the sexual relationship with one's partner. Information and counseling specific to ostomies can help greatly.

Estimates are that it may take up to a year to make a full and relatively comfortable adjustment to an ostomy.

Your primary physician as well as your surgeon are central in helping you anticipate and circumvent or resolve problems. Although most are grateful that their lives have been spared by ostomies, it is normal to experience difficulties in accepting the changes in one's body. Those who had active sex lives prior to ostomies usually continue to have them afterward, but inevitably there is a complex adjustment process, and you and your partner should not hesitate to seek help. Over a million people in the United States have had ostomies, and United Ostomy Clubs have been formed, which can offer a great deal of support. For information on the local chapter nearest you (there are more than 250 nationwide), contact the United Ostomy Association, 19772 MacArthur Blvd., Suite 200, Irvine, CA 92612-2405. *Sex, Courtship and the Ostomate* is a pamphlet available from the association.

RECTAL CANCER SURGERY

If a cancerous tumor is operable and is not in the lower two-thirds of the rectum, surgery can be done that not only permits normal bowel function but also allows normal sexual activity. However, if removal of the tumor requires removal of the rectum and anus, with a permanent colostomy, men may become totally impotent. The closeness of the male genital organs to the lower rectum leaves essential nerve fibers vulnerable to damage from such surgery. Women, on the other hand, maintain the capacity for sexual arousal and orgasm even after rectal surgery, since the essential nerves involved are farther removed from the surgical site.

IN SUMMARY

In general, for both men and women, the emotionally charged aspects of surgery and its effects on sexuality can be relatively short-lived *if* people spell out their fears and *if* their misconceptions are cleared up. Unfortunately, they often do not get the opportunity to do this. Doctors do not always take the time to explain procedures and answer questions, although counseling before surgery is extremely helpful in preventing anxiety and clarifying misunderstandings. After the operation, continued advice and emotional support from medical personnel, family, friends, and special organizations are crucial. Be sure to ask for help, and if you remain troubled, seek professional psychotherapy to work through your more complicated feelings.

Even with the best modern techniques, rates of recovery vary with the individual after surgery of any kind. Some people find their stamina or vitality reduced for some time, even though healing has been satisfactory. These are normal variations. You have no reason to worry if this happens to you, as long as your surgeon has assured you that your postoperative recovery is progressing as it should be. Once you are feeling entirely well again, your level of sexual activity is likely to return to normal. If sexual problems do occur, Viagra and other treatments are proving to be highly successful in many cases.

CHAPTER 7

❧❧❧

SEXUAL FITNESS

Sex is one of the great free and renewable pleasures of life. To get the most out of it, however, you should be in shape for it. Two powerful aphrodisiacs are a vigorous and well-cared-for body and a lively personality. Much can be done to preserve the functioning of both, although we shall be talking here specifically about your body. The overall formula for keeping in good health and preventing a multitude of problems is a simple one: no smoking, very moderate use of alcohol, control of blood pressure and weight, balanced nutrition, regular exercise, and adequate rest.

FITNESS FOR OLDER PEOPLE

It's never too early to start and always too soon to stop paying attention to your physical fitness. The enjoyment of sex is enhanced by keeping your body as healthy and pain-free as possible. Apart from visits to the doctor for a specific complaint, older men and women ideally should have a physical examination every year. Women should also have a gynecological examination every six months, particularly to check for breast and vaginal cancer. Bring any problems in sexual functioning to your doctor's attention at the time of these examinations, if not at a special appointment in between. The purpose of all this is to detect and treat physical problems in their early stages and to obtain medical guidance for a program of preventive health care, including exercise, nutrition, and rest.

EXERCISE

You're too busy to exercise? Don't even try this excuse. Although only one in four adults gets the minimum recommended moderate exercise of thirty minutes a day, many spend up to four hours daily watching television and surfing the Internet. Yet exercise at even modest levels will improve your physical appearance and increase your longevity—something that TV and the Web can't claim. Exercise is crucial for a healthy heart, arteries, and respiratory system, and has a relaxing effect on the nervous system. Studies indicate that bones maintain their size and strength better during aging if you exercise regularly. In addition, exercise can improve your sex life. The only bad news (but not new news) is that exercise requires discipline and a certain amount of work! Although we are improving our habits as a nation, many Americans do not exercise at all, and older people exercise less often than younger people. This is unfortunate, since the older you are, the more help your body needs from you. So plan to exercise on a routine and daily basis.

Physical fitness is a condition of looking and feeling good and having the necessary physical reserves to enjoy a range of interests, including sex. Fitness has two components. *Organic fitness* involves basic health, a well-nourished body as free as possible from disease or infirmity, with physical limitations compensated for to the greatest degree possible. *Dynamic fitness* means not simply freedom from disease but the full ability to move vigorously and energetically. This involves efficiency of heart and lungs, muscular strength and endurance, balance, flexibility, coordination, and agility.

To reach an optimum level in both components of fitness, you need to perform two distinct kinds of exercise: one to keep the body limber and supple and strengthen the muscles (stretching, flexing, and weight-bearing exercises), the other to increase endurance, enlarge heart capacity, and expand lung capacity (aerobic exercises).

To achieve a personal level of fitness, you should exercise aerobically for at least twenty to thirty continuous minutes three to five times a week, at about 70 percent of your age-adjusted maximum heart rate. To find your maximum rate, subtract your age from 220. For example, a sixty-year-old would subtract 60 from 220, which is 160. Seventy percent of 160 would equal 112 heartbeats a minute, or about 18 beats every ten seconds. For aerobic benefits, fast walking, swimming, cycling, cross-country skiing, and skating, all of which involve continual movement, are better than basketball, dance, handball, tennis, and racquetball, which involve intermittent movement. Be wary of jogging and fast action sports like racquetball, which can cause injury to the bones and joints.

Brisk walking is perhaps the best all-around exercise for older people, especially when it is accompanied by a regimen of stretching and weight lifting. The squeezing action of the leg muscles on the veins during walking helps promote the return of blood to the heart. Start out by walking rapidly until you begin to feel tired. Rest and walk back to your starting point. Keep doing this for progressively longer distances until you reach a reasonable goal, such as a walk of two to three miles a day, five days a week, for at least forty-five minutes each day. (This may take a year if you have previously been sedentary.) Eventually your ideal goal should be to walk five miles daily for five or six days a week. A pedometer is an easy way to keep track of the distance covered each day. Simply divide the number of steps you take by two in order to get the number of miles you have traveled. Ten thousand steps equal approximately five miles. (For weight loss, 15,000 steps or more are recommended—and remarkably effective!) Tests indicate that the Digi-walker brand of electronic pedometers is one of the most accurate. It is available for $19.95 plus $5 shipping and handling from the International Longevity Center, www.jimg@ilcusa.org.

As a supplement to a regular program of exercise, take advantage of any opportunity for physical move-ment—walking upstairs (rather than using escalators and elevators), doing chores, mowing the lawn, gardening—in short, bending, stretching, and moving as much as possible. But don't depend on these activities alone to keep you supple.

A growing number of exercise books are being written specifically for middle-aged and older people. For specific stretching, strengthening, endurance, bal-ance, and aerobic exercises, see the excellent exercise video (forty-eight minutes) and 100-page book avail-able for $7 from the National Institute on Aging titled *Exercise: A Guide from the National Institute on Aging*, November 2000 (Publication No. NIH 99-4258) with a forward by Senator John Glenn (Phone: 800-222-2225 to order). This exercise regimen is based on research funded by the NIA and "road-tested" on scores of older Americans.

If you have been unusually inactive or had any indication of possible heart disease, take a treadmill stress test (available in most hospitals) before jogging, swimming, and other more vigorous activities. Swimming is particularly useful for anyone with a joint disease like arthritis or orthopedic problems such as damaged knees or chronic backache. It is not recommended as the major physical activity to protect against osteoporosis, however, because, unlike walking, it is not weight bearing on the long bones of the body.

The use of a stationary bicycle or a treadmill is popular with older people because they are accessible in all kinds of weather, and, if you have one of them in your home, it requires no transportation to and from exercise periods. They also allow accurate measurement of the amount of exercise you are getting. However, if you use a bicycle at home, you must have good knees and no major orthopedic problems, and you must be strongly motivated to exercise alone.

Spa fitness centers, exercise resorts, and some of the better aerobic centers and health clubs that are proliferating in and near major cities have begun to pay more attention to the medical as well as the aesthetic and social aspects of exercise. Canyon Ranch, located in both Tucson, Arizona, and Lenox, Massachusetts, has developed well-run fitness programs in an all-around health-resort setting that includes an array of medical evaluations and treatments. Programs such as those found at the Duke University Diet and Fitness Center in Durham, North Carolina, are less spalike but highly regarded from a medical standpoint. The Pritikin Longevity Center located in Aventura, Florida, has expansive health evaluations and on-site programs that get people started on lifelong health regimens. The Dean Ornish Program, available in many medical settings, aims at preventing or treating heart disease through diet, stress management, exercise, and psychosocial support. All of these programs offer health education, individualized diet and exercise programs, and behavioral training to change old habits and take on new ones. Although they tend to be very expensive, they seldom cost more than one would spend on ship cruises and overseas tourism; they could be considered a vacation aimed at lifelong health.

Most spas and fitness centers today are coed, and men must be warned that they will usually not be able to achieve the same level of flexibility as most women. This is not a sign that they are not trying hard enough. It simply means that male and female bodies are different. On the other hand, men often have a natural advantage over women in exercises that emphasize strength. Ideally, both men and women should approach exercise noncompetitively. In fact, precisely because there are wide variations in physical performance and capacity, your own individual physical condition should determine the exercise appropriate for you and its level and pace. If you become temporarily ill or inactive, you will usually need to return to an earlier level of activity and slowly work your way back up. In all cases, avoid strenuous bursts of sudden activity when you are out of shape. We also recommend that you discuss your exercise program with your doctor and ask him or her to advise you.

Some people don't exercise out of the fear that it will provoke a heart attack. What they do not realize is that exercise reduces the risk of stroke or heart attack. Blood clots form when the blood is sluggish rather than when it is circulating vigorously. (This is why it is especially important to get up and move about on long airflights or stop and exercise during automobile trips.) A now-classic study of 17,000 middle-aged and older Harvard alumni over several years by Dr. Ralph Paffenbarger and colleagues, published in *The Journal of the American Medical Association*, July 27, 1984, found a greater risk of coronary heart disease among those who led sedentary lifestyles. As described in Chapter 3, people who have had heart attacks are usually placed on an exercise program by their physicians shortly after their initial recovery in order to reduce the possibility of another attack. Exercise is also valuable for preventing and treating hypertension, diabetes, and osteoporosis.

Exercising Your Trouble Spots

There are specific exercises that can greatly improve your appearance if they are undertaken on a regular basis.

A *protruding abdomen*, so common among older men, can be controlled by serious dieting, strenuous aerobics, and by regularly performing exercises which strengthen both the upper and lower abdominal muscles.

The upper abdomen is strengthened by exercises called *crunches*. To start, lie on your back on a thick rug or exercise mat on the floor. Bend your knees so that your feet rest flat on the floor. Put your hands behind your head. Use your upper abdominal muscles to raise your shoulders off the floor in a forward curling motion. Hold for a count of three. Then slowly lower your shoulders back to the floor again. Repeat this movement twenty times in one set. Start with one set per day, building up gradually to three to five sets per day. Take a rest of about one to two minutes between sets.

The lower abdomen is exercised further by *knee raises*. To start, lie flat on your back on the floor on a rug or exercise mat. Place your hands, palms down, under your buttocks. Bend your knees so that your feet are flat on the floor. Use your lower abdominal muscles to slowly raise your feet off the floor and bring your knees up to your chest. Then slowly bring your feet back to the floor to the starting position. Repeat as described for the upper abdominal crunches.

Improving *back muscles* will help your stomach muscles, as well as prevent or alleviate back pain. As much as 80 percent of backaches are due to muscle fatigue, weakness, and inactivity rather than slipped discs or arthritis. Lie on your back, squeeze your buttocks together, and tighten stomach muscles while flattening your back against the floor. Hold for a count of five, then relax. Repeat ten times. Swimming is also excellent for those with back problems.

In later years many women develop *weakened pelvic muscles*, which make them feel their vagina is losing its gripping ability. The Kegel exercises for women consist of contractions of the muscles of the pelvic floor, as though one were holding oneself back from urinating and defecating at the same time. It should be possible to feel the muscles tightening. Perform these exercises several times daily while in either a sitting or standing position. Hold the contraction for only a few seconds each time. The process must be repeated daily for at least one hundred contractions for the Kegel exercises to be truly effective.

Many women find the Kegel exercises difficult because they find it hard to focus on exercising the correct muscles. One helpful device women can use is the Femina Cone. When inserted into the vagina, the smooth plastic weighted cone will tend to slip out unless the proper muscles are contracted. This helps women learn which muscles to contract for Kegel exercises. For more information on Femina Cones, write Dacomed, Inc., 1701 East 79th St., Minneapolis, MN 55425.

When there is improved muscle tone as a result of using the Kegel exercises, the vaginal walls also then exert greater pressure on the penis. This is of particular value in those older couples where the man's penis has become somewhat smaller when erect and the woman's vagina larger, usually due to childbirth. Some women are able to use the Kegel movement in a rhythmic fashion during sexual intercourse, thus increasing both partners' satisfaction. The exercises also help to support the pelvic structure—the uterus, bladder, and rectum. Some physicians even prescribe Kegel exercises for men, to treat or prevent prostatitis.

Posture

The last word on posture is to stand tall (yes, your mother was right), although not in the ramrod posture popular in military training. Stand firmly on your two feet and then extend your head up as far as comfortably possible; the rest of the body, including the spine, will then tend to fall correctly in a relaxed alignment. It may require vigilance to remember this stance, especially if you are attempting to change years of bad posture habits. But the "stand tall" mind-set can be nurtured through yoga, such body therapies as the Alexander Method, and personal training with health professionals skilled in body mechanics and alignment.

For an easy and effective exercise to avoid "rounded" shoulders, stand in a doorway, place one hand on each side of the door frame at about the height of your shoulders, and with knees slightly bent, lean forward to stretch out the chest. Hold the position for ten seconds, and repeat five times daily.

NUTRITION

If you are over sixty, beware of poor nutrition and even malnutrition. You may protest, "That's absurd! I've always eaten a normal diet." Well, poor nutrition can creep up on you in later life. Medical and lay people alike share the illusion that the United States is the world's best-fed nation, but "overfed" is more accurate. Over 50 percent of adults are overweight. The United States has the highest percentage of overweight people in the world, and poor nutrition is widespread, even among those who eat large amounts of food.

This state of affairs is especially true when it comes to older people. There are many reasons for this, the most obvious being the cost of good-quality food and the lowered incomes of many people, especially women, as they grow older. But there are other, less obvious reasons. Social isolation and depression can cause people to lose their appetite and stop taking an interest in cooking; physical limitations may make shopping and preparing food difficult; loss of teeth or poor teeth interfere with eating solid foods; illnesses, alcoholism, and chronic diseases of many kinds can affect food consumption; and finally, poor eating habits may develop (snacking, the tea-and-toast syndrome, and use of junk food, "fast food," and convenience foods). Those who live alone are especially prone to neglect a proper diet—"It's too much bother to fix a meal for just one person."

What are the dangers of poor nutrition? You become more vulnerable to disease. You get fatigued more easily and lose your sense of well-being. You are also more likely to have emotional problems, among them depression, apathy, and anxiety. Age-related processes can be accelerated, and sexual interest and performance are often lowered. In other words, there are a host of reasons to eat well, aside from enjoying the taste of food itself.

How can you embark on a healthy, nutritious diet? A healthy diet includes three kinds of food groups—carbohydrates (cereals, breads, vegetables, fruits), proteins (meat, dairy products, eggs, fish, poultry, beans, nuts, and some grains), and fats (meat, dairy products, oils, nuts, and grains).

Carbohydrates, the complex starches and natural sugars in fruits, vegetables, and grains, are emerging as the healthiest foods overall, supplemented by poultry, fish, and low-fat and low-sugar dairy products. You should strictly limit your intake of red meat, any kind of animal or dairy fat, and, if you have high cholesterol, egg yolks. Refined carbohydrates are often the most tempting foods, and both sweet tooths, who love sugar, and people who find starchy foods irresistible may overload their diets with them. Refined starches, sugar, and other sweeteners fill the stomach, raise the blood sugar, lower the appetite, and lead to a false sense of well-being. Do not be deceived. *You must have some proteins every day for vitality and body-tissue repair.* If cost is a problem, learn more about preparing foods "from scratch" using low-cost proteins (dried skim milk, dried beans, cheaper cuts of meat, etc.). The home economics departments of high schools or colleges near you can offer advice, as will the U.S. Department of Agriculture. Write to the Superintendent of Documents, Government Printing Office, Washington, DC 20402, for nutrition information. In general, it is wise to cut down on desserts, pastries, fatty meats, gravies, beer, sweet wines, hard liquors, and soft drinks. Use heart-healthy oils, especially olive and canola oils, which are good sources of monounsaturated fatty acids. Try to eliminate or greatly reduce use of butter, lard, cream, and most margarines.

If you happen to be overweight and need to diet, reliable authors on this topic are Jane Brody of *The New York Times*, Dean Ornish, M.D., and Robert Pritikin. Look for their latest books. Also see *The Omega Diet*, by Artemis Simopoulous, M.D. and Jo Robinson.

Avoid crash and fad diets since they can harm your health and your appearance. Develop food habits you can live with comfortably, in good health, while still losing weight. Supplementing a sensible weight-loss diet with regular aerobic exercise is the surest way to lose weight and keep that weight off. Diet clubs such as TOPS, Weight Watchers, Jenny Craig, and Overeaters Anonymous, or self-organized dieting clubs can make it easier for people with persistent weight problems to lose pounds.

Diets aimed at the prevention of disease are important far before age sixty. We know a good deal, for example, about diet and the prevention and control of heart disease. The earliest of the heart disease prevention diets is the Prudent Man's Diet, devised by Dr. Norman Jolliffe in 1957. This was a balanced, low-calorie diet that called for a total of 2,400 calories a day (compared to the American male's average of 3,200), with no more than 30 percent fat, a cholesterol limit of 300 milligrams a day (roughly the amount in one egg), moderate protein, increased complex carbohydrates such as vegetables and fruits, and a reduction of salt.

Epidemiological cross-national data exist that relate health and longevity with even lower-fat diets (e.g., in China, only 10 percent of calories in the daily diet are in the form of fat). The Pritikin and Ornish diets mentioned earlier call for individuals to eat only 10 percent of daily calories in fat. However, the American Heart Association recommends a maximum of 30 percent. In truth it is not the amount of fat per se but rather the types of fats to be avoided, specifically saturated and trans-fats. The new FDA food labeling system will help you in calculating the specific fat content of foods. You can also obtain recipes and cooking advice from your local heart association or from the American Heart Association, 205 East 42nd Street, New York, NY 10017.

To help you become more aware about the dangers

and benefits of cholesterol, look at the following information:

- •The average blood cholesterol for all Americans today is 210 milligrams (per deciliter of blood). For older people, a cholesterol level of 240 to 260 milligrams indicates moderate risk of heart attack, while levels above 260 milligrams are at high risk. Aim for a level between 160 and 200.
- A specific subfraction of high-density lipoprotein cholesterol, called HDL_2, may actually protect against heart attack. Recent studies indicate that an extended program of regular aerobic exercise raises HDL_2.
- Fatty fish, such as salmon and mackerel, and monounsaturated fats, such as olive oil, may have cholesterol-lowering effects.
- Nearly all clinical trials of the effects of cholesterol lowering have focused on middle-aged men. We know less about women and even less about older persons. Some feel that those who are very old and frail should not restrict their cholesterol intake because of the risk of not eating enough to meet their caloric and nutritional needs.

Other specific nutritional tips for those of you who are older:

- Go easy on salt, since you are more susceptible to high blood pressure.
- Bulk in your diet is very important for diges-
  tion. This is true for all older people but
  especially for those who are dieting to lose
  weight. Doctors used to prescribe low-residue
  (limited-bulk) diets for older people with
  bowel problems, but now just the opposite is
  generally true. Bulk can be obtained by eating
  fruits and vegetables (complex carbohydrates) like raw celery, apples, and carrots, as
  well as whole-grain bread and cereals. Bran
  cereal is also a good choice. If you want lots of
  bulk at low cost, buy coarse bran (local
  health-food stores usually carry it) for a few
  cents a pound. If you don't live near a health-
  food store, get a mail-order health-food cata-
  log. Coarse bran tastes like a cross between
  babies' pabulum and sawdust (in other
  words—not so good!), but if you take several
  teaspoonfuls in between swallows of fruit
  juice at each meal or a larger amount on your
  breakfast cereal daily, you will be taking an
  important step in promoting good bowel action and preventing diverticulosis, certain
  kinds of constipation, and other bowel problems. Bran is *far* better for you than laxatives.
  And the complex carbohydrates may be even
  better.

- Try to avoid getting into the habit of taking laxatives, which can in fact induce habitual constipation. As we have noted, a good diet with plenty of bulk, plenty of exercise, and plenty of fluids (eight glasses a day) are the best ways to prevent constipation. If you do need an occasional laxative, many doctors feel that milk of magnesia is preferable to mineral oil, which tends to reduce the absorption of fat-soluble vitamins.
- "Indigestion" from eating fried foods may mean gallstones, so consult your doctor. Some liver specialists believe that a low-fat diet can help prevent the formation of gallstones.
- Gout, arthritis, diabetes, and a number of other diseases that can directly affect your sex life as well as your general health may require a special diet prescribed by your doctor.
- Many older people probably would benefit from taking a standard vitamin-and-mineral supplement daily. For the average healthy individual, a multivitamin should contain no more than 100 to 150 percent of the U.S. Recommended Daily Allowance (RDA) for any one nutrient. Ordinarily iron is not a necessary supplement, since excess iron can adversely affect the heart. After the menopause, women need no more iron than men do.
- Anemia (reduced hemoglobin and/or red

blood cells) may occur when your diet is inadequate in iron and protein. Foods containing iron are lean meats, dark green leafy vegetables, and whole grain and enriched breads and cereals. Altering your diet to provide for the adequate amounts of iron and protein is more economical and just as effective as the highly advertised vitamin-and-mineral preparations. (Remember: Your anemia should be evaluated by your doctor.)

- Osteoporosis, a common disorder, is due to a gradual loss of calcium from the bones, and its development is accelerated in women by the onset of menopause. Wrist and hip fractures and deformities such as a hump on the back may develop. High protein and salt intake, cigarette smoking, heavy caffeine and alcohol intake, lack of exercise, and a family history of osteoporosis all work toward increasing the risk of osteoporosis. The disorder may be slowed in some by adequate nutrition and exercise, although specific recommendations for doing so are still under debate. For example, opinions differ on the significance of calcium intake, with some believing that an excess of protein in the diet may be even more significant than insufficient calcium in the development of osteoporosis. Currently estrogen replacement therapy is considered the most effective preventative treatment, but because of its possible risks, such therapy should be individualized by you and your doctor (see Chapter 2). Persons who already have osteoporosis may be better treated with one of a new class of drugs called bisphosphonates, which include alendronate and risedronate.

Efforts to prevent osteoporosis should begin in childhood and youth, with an emphasis on exercise, calcium intake, and avoidance of smoking. But you can still help to slow or delay osteoporosis starting in your middle years by increasing your calcium to an adequate intake of 1,000 milligrams before menopause and 1,500 milligrams after it. (The average intake of adult women is 450 to 500 milligrams a day—far too low.) About five eight-ounce glasses of skim milk (to avoid fat intake) would supply 1,500 milligrams of calcium. If you don't like milk or it does not agree with you, you should take calcium supplements containing carbonate. However, Tums, a good source of calcium carbonate, causes constipation for some. An alternative is orange juice fortified with calcium citrate. Other good sources of calcium include such foods as yogurt, hard cheese (especially Parmesan and Swiss—but do use these sparingly), canned salmon and sardines (you should eat the bones, too), kidney and pinto beans, bean curd, oysters, and collard, turnip, and mustard greens.

If you are postmenopausal, be careful not to take

more than the recommended amount of 1,500 milligrams; calcium in larger doses can have harmful effects. Those of you taking additional estrogen can scale back to a normal premenopausal dosage of 1,000 milligrams daily. Moreover, those with a tendency to develop kidney stones, ulcers, or other digestive disorders may react adversely to high calcium intake.

Hip fractures can also occur as a result of a condition called sarcopenia, namely the loss of muscle mass, muscle quality, and strength. Sarcopenia is caused by inactivity. Prevention and treatment involve weight-bearing exercises and exercises to improve balance.

Further tips on nutrition:

- Large doses of vitamin E have been recommended for a variety of disorders, including sterility and vascular diseases, and for retarding aging processes, curing impotence, and healing wounds and burns. There is as yet no definitive scientific evidence for these claims, but anecdotal evidence for certain conditions is widespread. Controlled studies are underway to see if vitamin E slows the progression or prevents Alzheimer's Disease. The recommended daily allowance for women is 20 to 25 international units (IU) and for men 30 IU, although up to 400 IU per day is not thought to be harmful.
- In general, be prudent about taking over-the-

counter medications widely advertised on television and radio; they are sometimes valueless, often costly, and on occasion—especially if you take them in large quantities or combine them—hazardous. An office visit to your doctor may prove less expensive as well as better for your health than self-diagnosis and self-administered remedies for a physical complaint.

- It is a common belief that people need fewer calories as they grow older. One source claims that your body will require 10 percent fewer calories between ages thirty-five and fifty-five than when you were under thirty-five, 16 percent fewer between ages fifty-five and seventy-five, and 1 percent fewer calories per year for every year over seventy-five. We are not totally convinced of this. We suspect that this theory is based on the fact that many older people become less active and fail to work or exercise their bodies, and that caloric needs are a function of activity and not of age. (Some inactivity is of course related to physical ailments, but much more is simply lack of motivation and inertia.) The older you get, the more temptation you will feel to take it easy. Remember the maxim "Most people don't wear out, they rust out." Lack of movement leads to poor appetite, which in turn leads to fatigue and a vicious cycle.

- Experts tend to believe that it is harder to lose weight as we grow older, and some say this is especially true for women. Therefore, it is critical to practice a lifelong pattern of prudent eating and regular exercise, with perhaps even an increase in the amount of time and effort spent in exercising as you grow older.
- If you make your evening meal relatively light, you will find that you feel and sleep better. (Breakfast is the best time to eat heartily.) Cutting down on food and alcohol intake before bed is also conducive to better sex. If you do find yourself having a heavy evening meal, it would be best to postpone lovemaking for a few hours to avoid unnecessary strain on the heart and other organs.

REST

A rested body enhances sexual desire, improves sexual performance, and contributes to general health and well-being. Contrary to general opinion, as you grow older you will need as much sleep as when you were younger, or maybe even more. You may, however, notice changes in your sleep patterns. Studies show that older people seem to experience less deep or delta sleep (the period of dreamless oblivion), becoming lighter sleepers, with more frequent awakenings. In addition, depression, anxiety, grief, loneliness, and lack of exercise can affect both sleep patterns and depth of sleep. Early morning awakening is more common among the inactive, the depressed, those who go to bed early, and those who frequently take long naps during the day.

Get seven or more hours of sleep a night, according to your own personal needs. The amount of sleep needed varies from person to person, and you will find you need more sleep if you have physical health problems. If this applies to you, take one or more brief naps or rest breaks during the day, but limit total naptime to sixty minutes or less to avoid interfering with nighttime rest.

If insomnia strikes, don't panic. To be your most receptive for sleep, avoid caffeine drinks such as coffee, tea, and colas before bedtime—or better yet, after midday—since they can keep you awake. Drinking decaffeinated coffee is preferable, although some report that even the minimal amount of caffeine it contains can keep them awake. To get psychologically ready for sleep, you may want to establish these simple rituals: warm baths, firm and comfortable bed and pillows, back massage by a partner, reading a book, watching TV, or listening to music. Often warm milk, herbal tea, or soothing talks with your partner or an understanding friend can comfort and relax you. Exercise, too, can have a positive effect on sleep if completed early enough in the day, particularly if it has been performed on a regular basis for at least two months. But avoid exercising for two hours before bedtime, so that insomnia does not develop from the recent stimulation of your body.

Bedtime is a time when your defenses against anxiety, anger, and other emotions are lowered. If these emotions routinely create troubled sleep or insomnia, you may find that psychotherapy or some other form of counseling may help. Go out of your way to avoid nonprescription sleep remedies; they are expensive and, on the whole, useless. Eventually your body will become tired enough to sleep all by itself! For occasional insomnia, one or two aspirin or Tylenol (including Tylenol PM) before bed are helpful for some people. We don't recommend sleeping pills (hypnotics) unless you are in pain or great physical or emotional discomfort; they can be habit-forming and may cause adverse side effects, including, paradoxically, the perpetuation of insomnia. (However, for occasional use, Ambien and Sonata have the fewest problems.) If you do use sleeping pills, ensure that your use of them is evaluated by your physician on an ongoing basis—these prescriptions should not be automatically renewed.

Engaging in active, pleasurable sexual activity, including sexual self-stimulation, is an excellent way of inducing sleep. The effect is strongest when you have an orgasm, but even without it you will find that such activity is usually mildly relaxing.

When it comes to serious sleep disturbances and disorders, contact your physician. You may be able to find specialists in sleep disorders in your area by contacting the National Sleep Foundation, 1522 K Street NW, Suite 500, Washington, DC, 20005.

HEARING PROBLEMS

One out of every four older people has a hearing impairment. For various reasons—among them embarrassment, pride, and a psychological determination to deny the fact—a surprising number of people refuse to use hearing aids even when these aids will help. Not all hearing impairments can be improved by wearing a hearing aid, but only an audiologist (a specialist trained in a program accredited by the American Speech and Hearing Association) or an otologist or otolaryngologist (doctors specifically trained to treat ear disorders) can determine this; if you suspect you have some hearing loss, you should consult with one of these specialists. Remember, too, that hearing impairments tend to develop gradually, so you may be unaware this is happening to you. If you find yourself frequently missing parts of ordinary conversation around you or have trouble making out the dialogue when you go to the movies, it is a good idea to have your hearing checked.

Impaired hearing isolates you from society far more than you realize. Present-day hearing aids are much less conspicuous, disfiguring, and cumbersome than they used to be, and observers are very likely to be matter-of-fact about them. If yours is the type of loss that can be compensated for by the use of a hearing aid, do not let personal inhibitions stop you from using one! You will realize how much you have been missing only after your hearing improves.

It will take time for you to accustom yourself to a hearing aid, so be prepared for an adjustment period; stick with it despite your initial discomfort, and thereafter always use your aid whenever you are with another person.

Be very careful to deal only with a responsible supplier. This is a field full of high-pressure door-to-door salesmen offering "low" prices, "easy" installment payments, and defective or shoddy equipment. It is important that you be properly tested and fitted with an aid of good quality, one that is appropriate to your needs.

People who have the kind of hearing loss that cannot be helped by a hearing aid *must* be frank with friends and intimates. It is unlikely that they will find your disclosure embarrassing; the awkwardness is more likely to be on your side. Sit close to your companion so you can hear what is being said and speak up when you do not. It is only when you attempt to conceal a hearing impairment that problems are likely to arise.

SKIN CARE FOR MEN AND WOMEN

Ideally, prevention of skin problems should begin in the early years for both men and women, but good skin care can help at *any* time in life. Skin can be damaged by too much sun or wind and by malnutrition, excess alcohol or tobacco (nicotine), diseases, depression, drugs, and anxiety. Overexposure to the sun causes more premature aging—particularly in Caucasians—than any other factor. Sunbathing and working or playing out-of-doors unprotected for long periods of time are the major culprits. They can result in permanent skin damage affecting both the outer and inner layers of skin, causing loss of water and elasticity, deep wrinkles, and grooves. Prolonged exposure to very cold weather, overheated rooms with minimal humidity, and air conditioning in warm climates can deplete the moisture in the skin, making it look lined. Electric blankets left on all night can dry the body skin. Various kinds of air pollution can be damaging as well. Poor nutrition, whether vitamin deficiencies or unbalanced diets, can cause dry, scaly, and inelastic skin. Sagging skin sometimes follows too rapid weight loss. Anxiety, depression, and tension also speed up the appearance of aging. Cigarette smoking can cause wrinkles to appear sooner than they normally would, since nicotine narrows the small capillaries and cuts down the supply of blood bringing nourishment and oxygen to the skin. The result, often called "smoker's face," includes deep vertical wrinkles from the corners of lips or eyes, facial gauntness, and a grayish pallor.

Even with the best preventive care, the human face begins to acquire noticeable lines and wrinkles around the age of forty. At this time there is a gradual and permanent loss of elasticity in both the skin and the underlying tissue. Wrinkles per se should not become an obsessive concern; looking your age does not mean looking unattractive. But all of us—even those not enmeshed in the cult of youth—want to look our best. Just don't waste your money on "wrinkle removers" and other gimmicks "guaranteed" to make you look younger; anything that keeps the skin moist will help to slow down the appearance of aging.

Here is a simple regimen that you can follow to take care of your skin. The first step involves thoroughly cleansing the face and neck. Many older people can tolerate a mild, super fatted soap like Dove if it is used quickly and rinsed off completely. Neutrogena, which is much more expensive than many common soaps, is also a possibility, or a rinsable cleanser, which combines cream and a small amount of soap in lotion form. (Creams and oils used alone are difficult to remove, so the skin is never completely cleansed.) After cleansing and a thorough rinsing with warm water, pat your face dry and immediately protect it with a light moisturizer by day or a heavier oily cream for night while the skin still holds the moisture absorbed from the rinse. Most inexpensive creams like Pond's work as well as the expensive ones. Protect the skin on your body against drying by using a body lotion immediately after a bath or shower when the skin has absorbed moisture.

Electric facial saunas dry out the skin. The face should really not be massaged, but if you must do it, never stretch or pull the skin in any downward direction. Various chemical processes and dermabrasion (removal of the tissues of the outer skin layer with a rotating wire brush) can be dangerous unless done by skilled operators. They are also expensive. Plastic surgery (face-lifts) for both men and women can correct severe skin sagging, but they, too, are expensive, and good results last only three to five years. The best skin care advice we have for you is sunscreen protection, sensible cleansing, good diet, rest and lack of tension, and avoidance of cigarette smoking and excess alcohol.

PRACTICAL STRATEGIES FOR CREATING YOUR HEALTHIER LIFESTYLE*

You will be more likely to be successful in establishing a healthier lifestyle if you plan the changes and then monitor your progress regularly. A new behavior is relatively easy to introduce, but much harder to maintain. The following is a list of steps to follow:

- Establish a goal and make a contract with yourself. The three most vital areas to target are nutrition, tobacco cessation, and physical exercise.
- Personalize your program to address special needs or health risks, such as diabetes, high blood pressure, or high cholesterol.
- Find convenient and inexpensive ways to achieve your goals.
- Self-monitor your efforts. If your goal is weight loss, write down exactly what you eat. If your goal is to become more physically

*Reprinted with permission from *Maintaining Healthy Lifestyles: A Lifetime of Choices*. New York: The International Longevity Center, December 1999.

fit, wear an electronic-based pedometer (see page 188) to clock the number of steps you take in a given day, whether you walk, jog, or run.

- Build healthy habits and activities around your schedule. Establish routines that are environment-friendly, at the workplace, school, and home.
- Find a role model to emulate in adopting a healthier lifestyle.
- Establish a peer-support system. Mutual support encourages compliance, whether it is a partner, a club, or family members.
- Establish a professional-support system with a physician or fitness trainer who can offer guidance and support.

CHAPTER 8

❧ ❧

COMMON EMOTIONAL PROBLEMS WITH SEX

Upsetting events in our life—the death of a loved one, retirement, relationship conflicts, or simply too much stress and worry—can cause sexual problems. And growing older itself can be frightening, especially if you don't know what to expect or how to handle it. Your early life experiences and society's attitudes also have an impact on how you handle your sexuality. Baby boomers approaching their sixties will have different attitudes from people already in their sixties, seventies, and beyond. Let's delve a little deeper into these areas.

PERSONAL ANXIETIES

A major emotional problem older men face is the *fear* of sexual impotence. While some men have to deal with actual potency problems, they are usually temporary. In fact, *erectile difficulties occur occasionally in nearly all men of all ages* for a variety of reasons—among them fatigue, tension, illnesses, and excessive drinking. In most cases potency returns by itself without specific treatment when the causative physical or emotional condition is reversed. In later life, however, certain men do begin to have chronic difficulty in obtaining and maintaining an erection or find that their capacity for sexual intercourse is greatly diminished or disappears completely. We discussed the possible organic causes of potency problems in Chapters 3 and 5, but it is unwise to overlook the fact that many such difficulties can also have psychological foundations. The sexual organs are a barometer of a man's feelings and quickly reflect his state of mind and current life situation. In fact, the nerve connections that control the penis are extremely sensitive to emotions. Anxiety, fear, depression, and anger are the primary feelings that can cause a man to lose an erection rapidly—or fail to achieve one in the first place. So a disturbance in sexual functioning is often one of the first indications of unusual stress or emotional problems.

Men who do not know about the *normal* physiological changes in their sexual behavior that come with aging may believe falsely that they are becoming impotent. The expectation of high performance, which is taught to males from childhood on through constant emphasis on competition and winning, leads many men to overemphasize the physical-performance aspect of their sexuality. They become focused on erections and ejaculations rather than on recognizing their feelings. This makes impotence or even its threat greatly upsetting. Thus, the very *fear* of impotence can *cause* potency problems. The harder a man tries to have an erection, the less likely he is to succeed. Erectile difficulties do not respond to willpower and force. And if they are truly transitory, they are much more likely to improve with relaxation and freedom from pressure.

Unresponsive sexual partners can threaten men and lead to erectile problems. A woman's disinterest or perfunctory acquiescence is very likely to affect her partner. Women may also become impatient or demanding and make a transitory potency problem more severe. Some even find erectile problems threatening to their own self-esteem and react with hostility or hurt; they see it as a sign of disinterest in them or a failure on their part to be sexually attractive.

Emotional and physical fatigue, boredom with routine lovemaking, overwork, and worries about family or finances can all affect potency. Erectile problems are often one of the first symptoms of depression. Disappointment, sadness, and grief over personal losses can be factors. So can resentfulness and irritation.

Sometimes erectile problems result from an unrecognized fear of death or injury. Fred, a businessman and retired army officer, had been a vigorous and sexually active man until he suffered a coronary attack at age seventy-two. After the attack he was unable to have an erection. It took many sessions with a psychiatrist to help him recognize that his *fear* of sexual activity triggering another coronary was the reason he did not allow himself to have an erection. His doctors suggested a provisional program of exercise, including sex that would not jeopardize his heart. As Fred's anxiety lessened through psychotherapeutic counseling, and his sense of well-being increased as a result of his physical fitness program, his sexual ability returned.

A sudden attack of difficulties with potency is likely to be the result of some unusual stress and, once the stress is relieved, will usually abate. Even if you've experienced a lack of potency for quite some time, all you may need to overcome your condition might be information and reassurance from a doctor or professional counselor. If you find problems still persist, however, you may require a comprehensive medical evaluation and more extended psychotherapy and/or sexual counseling. Through this all, it is important to recognize that your partner's support plays a critical role in overcoming your problem.

Women are somewhat less subject to the fear of

sexual dysfunction in later life than men are, mainly because they do not have to worry about erection. Except for possible menopausal changes, the normal physical changes that accompany aging interfere very little with a woman's sexual ability. Unlike most men, women can perform the sexual act even when they are emotionally upset or uninterested. While they may not enjoy lovemaking or have an orgasm in these situations, they are physically capable of having intercourse. (One worry women may have is about orgasmic capacity, much as men are concerned about erection and ejaculatory capacity.) Indeed, in later life some women become more relaxed about sex and come to enjoy it more, once menopause has freed them from their fear of unwanted pregnancies. Their lives may also become less pressured, their responsibilities diminishing after their children leave home; in this way the "empty nest" frequently becomes a welcome event rather than a problem.

But women can and do have other problems. Especially in the oldest age groups, men and women grew up believing that "nice" women were not interested in sex and indeed found it distasteful. Women were traditionally admonished or conditioned to be passive, resigned, and accepting; it was only "loose" women who gave themselves to the pleasures of sex or sought it. Women may remember being taught by their mothers and grandmothers that sex was simply a duty. Men were the pursuers, women were reluctant and pursued. Such ingrained attitudes interfere with developing close relationships in which both partners openly share in the enjoyment of sex. If this has been your experience, speak frankly about these issues with your partner, to clear up these antiquated assumptions. If you find it necessary, seek professional help.

The most profound emotional and sexual difficulties older women face revolve around the possibility of finding themselves alone—widowed, divorced, separated, or single—as they grow older. Their lives are affected by one major fact: there are not enough men to go around. In the United States in 1998 there were 13.5 million men aged sixty-five or over, and 18.6 million women. This disparity increases year by year as time passes, for two reasons. First, women outlive men by an average of seven years. (In 1998 life expectancy from birth was 79.5 years for females and 73.8 years for males, according to the Census Bureau.) Second, women marry men an average of three years older than themselves. And in 1998, of the 18.6 million women over sixty-five, 8.5 million were widowed (compared to only 2 million widowed men) and 2.2 million were divorced or single. This all adds up to the fact that nearly 60 percent of older women are on their own, a challenging fact when one considers that they, more than any younger group, were raised from childhood to consider themselves dependent on men. Research efforts to understand and eliminate the life-expectancy differential between men and women are increasing, bringing hope for more balance in the future.

THE "OLD-PERSON" TRAP

Even when their physical and mental health is excellent, men and women in their fifties, sixties, and seventies sometimes exhibit an old-man or old-woman act, as though they were tottering invalids on their last legs. They have a rigid, stereotyped, desexualized image of what an older person *should* be, and play the role with stubborn determination. Playing the "old-person act" allows them to avoid responsibility toward themselves and others and to evoke sympathy. It can be a symbol of a perverse reluctance to "grow up" into a mature old age, or it can be simply a sign of demoralization and giving up.

Many simply decide their sexual ability is gone and arbitrarily declare themselves to be sexually incapacitated. They typically refuse to discuss the issue with their partner or to even consider possible remedies. What lies behind these actions is an attempt to avoid any type of anxiety about sex or a sexual relationship.

Such was the case with Paul, age seventy-two, a classic example of someone playing the old-person act. He shuffled along with his head bent and body slouched—in spite of the fact that he was in perfect health. He also had both a supportive wife and family, and was financially secure. So why *was* he acting this way? Paul denied that he was doing anything, but his wife claimed it was because he was angry and depressed at growing old. Paul didn't try to help himself overcome this attitude. The outcome? His wife ended up losing respect for him, and eventually her sexual interest in him waned.

Many believe they have become ugly and undesirable and begin to hate the way they look as a result of the aging process. They make frantic attempts to appear young, and end up becoming depressed at the futility of altering their appearance significantly. This was how Marlena felt. Whenever she looked in the mirror she could see the thickening in her thighs. She tried to control her eating, but even after she lost ten pounds, her legs failed to regain their former shape. She tried many supposed cures and embarked on a low-impact aerobics course. Nothing helped. It got to the point that Marlena made her partner Jim turn off the lights whenever they made love. She simply could not believe that he would be interested in her if he saw how she "truly" looked.

Another variation of this kind of self-hatred is found in those who look into the mirror and insist that what they see "is not the real me." They may decide that their only true self is interior, and refuse to accept or identify with their physical characteristics. It may take some time, but they must eventually accept the realities of change.

Sometimes older people angrily respond to their own sexual and social deprivation with hostility toward those who are younger. Everyone has heard bitter threats such as "You'll see what it's like when *you're* old" or "Wait until you reach *my* age—you won't be so smart." They might even offer self-righteous criticism of the sexuality of their own contemporaries as well as of the young.

It is vital that you recognize that you *can* make a self-fulfilling prophecy of sexual failure. Don't let yourself be overwhelmed and demoralized by the unattractive picture society draws of late life, so that you literally give up without trying, or guarantee your own failure when you do try. *To anticipate failure is to cause it to happen.* If you think you are unattractive, you tend to become so. If you believe you are sexually ineligible, you are likely to hide from those opportunities that might lead to social and sexual encounters.

So how can you avoid the old-person trap? One of the best cures is to find lively and attractive older persons with whom you can associate and identify. They provide invaluable role models when you are just beginning to search out satisfying ways to live your own life. Talk to them, ask their advice, and try on new behaviors. And when you are ready, take on the responsibility of being a role model to others.

SEXUAL GUILT AND SHAME

Sexual guilt and shame play a role in many people's reaction to sex. These feelings derive from childhood and family experiences, and from the sexual searchings of childhood, which can so often be confusing and disturbing. Numbers of people past sixty are likely to have been treated to more than their share of misinformation, made to feel guilty about childhood sexual stirrings they sensed, and given few chances to get satisfying answers to their questions—if they dared ask them in the first place. Oddly enough, American culture still has not found a way to address sexuality and the normal expression of it—looking, feeling, talking, touching—in a straightforward and accepting manner for the young.

Not so very long ago, masturbation itself was strictly forbidden. The Victorians even invented a grotesque array of mechanical devices to make certain that children, both boys and girls, would not be able to stimulate themselves. Our grandparents were likely to have warned our parents that masturbation could cause feeblemindedness or madness; it could "use up the life juices," weaken the body and shorten the life span, and make one nervous, distracted, and high-strung. Dark circles under the eyes were alleged indications of secret masturbation, and a grisly folklore sprang up in which hands withered and fell off if they were used in sexual stimulation. Even today, masturbation is seldom treated as a normal and even enjoyable activity.

An important misassumption that many older men still have from their youth is that "too much" sexual activity reduces potency and lowers semen "reserves." The belief that semen must be conserved is sheer nonsense, because it is constantly produced—yet as late as 1945 the *Boy Scout Manual* warned youths not to "waste vital fluids."

For older men and women (certainly for those over seventy) the greater part of their procreative years occurred before birth control techniques were as sophisticated, reliable, and freely available as they are today. As a result, spontaneous sexual enjoyment was often hampered by the fear of pregnancy and justified fears of venereal disease, for which effective drugs had not yet been devised. Many traditional religious teachings also imposed psychological inhibitions on sexuality.

These teachings still exert an influence on older people today. A woman in her seventies wrote:

> I feel guilty about having sexual relations with a man I'm not married to. Carl and I are both widowed, in our early seventies, and have known each other for thirty years. Every month we spend a few days at each other's home.
>
> Carl says we shouldn't feel guilty at our age and that he would like to marry me. Al-

though I enjoy our relationship, I don't want to remarry. I've been widowed twice, most recently four years ago. Do you see any harm in my relationship with Carl?

Often it is hard for older people to give themselves freely to sexual expression. It is not easy to overcome ingrained guilt and shame even when your better judgment tells you that sexuality need no longer be considered evil or dangerous (keeping in mind, of course, that if you are not in a strictly monogamous relationship you must practice "safe sex" as a precaution against AIDS [See Chapter 4]). Thinking through your own childhood and early adult experiences may help you understand your present feelings better. Such feelings may initially be difficult to resolve, but remember once again that sexual problems, whether caused by personal or by social factors, are rarely insurmountable if approached with determination and accurate information. (A sense of humor about sex is a godsend as well.)

PROBLEMS BETWEEN PARTNERS

If you are experiencing problems in your relationship with your sexual partner, these can very quickly affect your sexual functioning. An angry, bored, or otherwise unresponsive partner can lead to potency problems for men and sexual disinterest or lack of response for women.

Low sexual interest rather than potency per se may be a central problem for many men. Dr. Joseph LoPiccolo, a well-respected expert in the field of sexual behavior, believes that a chronic low sex drive is much more common among men than was previously thought. He describes most of this as psychologically based, ranging from the effects of feeling overwhelmed by life events to fears of intimacy.

Women, according to Dr. LoPiccolo, are becoming more likely to question male performance and behavior and are often the ones who will initiate treatment for the male with low sexual interest. But women themselves may exhibit the symptoms. Called by the pejorative term "frigidity," this behavior used to be interpreted as fear and active resistance to sexuality, but now it is more often viewed as low sexual desire and lack of responsiveness.

Although a lack of sexual desire can be a comfortable way of life for some, more often it troubles at least one partner. Sex therapists note that a growing proportion of their patients seek help for what is currently called "inhibited sexual desire." While occasional and short-lived lack of sexual desire is commonplace and reversible, if it is long lasting, it can be one of the most difficult and intractable of sexual symptoms. For those who wish to change, a combination of sex therapy, psychotherapy, and marriage counseling over an extended period of time may prove to be the most beneficial.

Others experience sexual desire but find that the physical responsiveness is absent. This manifests itself as potency problems in men and failure to lubricate and reach orgasm in women. Its causes can encompass a range of emotions from depression, grief, and stress to anxiety, fear, and anger. Ordinarily the sexual response returns when the underlying emotions are resolved or improved. But such psychologically based symptoms, whatever their original emotional cause, can also quickly create performance anxiety and continued sexual problems if people are intimidated, embarrassed, or frightened by the changes in their sexual functioning. This is particularly true of men, for whom "performance" carries great importance.

The first step in self-treatment is for both you and your partner to relax and assume that sexual functioning is likely to improve once emotional equilibrium is restored. Kindness and consideration toward each other and a lack of psychological pressure are crucial for recovery. It is important to remember that a sexual response cannot be willed. It is most likely to occur when a person is rested, relaxed, and in a positive mood, and enjoying a good relationship with his or her partner.

An important way of inducing arousal is through physical stimulation. You should first involve the body as a whole and later focus on the genitals. Masters and Johnson initiated a three-stage method of "sensate focus," which is now used by many sex therapists to teach people to relax and slowly move each other into a state of sexual arousal that eventually results in an orgasm. The stages are, first, to embark step-by-step on a nongenital "pleasuring" of your partner's body by touching and caressing it; second, to touch and caress the genitals, stopping short of actual sex; and third, to engage in nondemanding sexual intercourse where the goal is pleasure rather than performance.

Premature ejaculation also is a fairly common problem, affecting 15 to 20 percent of American men, according to Masters and Johnson. While occasional and temporary premature ejaculation happens to most men from time to time (especially when they have had infrequent sex or are unusually aroused), it usually disappears by itself as circumstances change. However, persistent premature ejaculation is another matter. It does not tend to develop for the first time in the mid or later years but usually begins early on, and it may well continue into later life. Fortunately it is often responsive to treatment.

Reassurance is the first step to try, along with making certain there are regular opportunities for sexual outlet.

If these efforts are not enough, a highly successful method has been developed by Masters and Johnson—the "squeeze" technique—in which the woman applies pressure to the head of her partner's erect penis in the following manner: She puts her thumb against the underside of the penis and her index and middle fingers opposite the thumb on either side of the ridge of tissue that separates the head of the penis from the shaft. She then gently presses all three fingers together (her partner can tell her how strongly to squeeze) for a few seconds. This causes the man to lose his urge to ejaculate but allows the couple to continue lovemaking. By alternating the squeezing with sex play, a couple may delay ejaculation until they are ready for a climax. A more detailed description of this technique appears in *Masters and Johnson on Sex and Human Loving* (Little, Brown and Co., 1986).

There is also the "stop-start" technique, which is perhaps the most frequent approach used. It refers to stopping genital stimulation until the urge to ejaculate disappears—at which time stimulation is resumed again. If these techniques fail to work, you may find psychotherapy helpful. In addition, you may find that premature ejaculation may become less of a problem as a man grows older, simply because some of the urgency to ejaculate diminishes.

CHANGES OVER TIME

Role changes over time can also cause disruptions in sexual behavior. One partner may alter his or her level of assertiveness, affecting the original emotional or power balance between the two. We sometimes see relationships in which the man has assumed a predominantly fatherly, protective role toward his more dependent partner. If he becomes sick and needs her care, serious problems, including sexual difficulties, can arise. The woman, who has always been babied, can become petulant, dissatisfied, or simply unable or unwilling to play a giving and responsible role. A variant of this is the hypochondriacal man—the worrywart—involved with an independent and caretaking woman who becomes ill. When she cannot mother her partner, the equilibrium in which they had functioned for so long is upset as well.

Most typically, women gradually become more assertive and men more nurturant as they grow older—in essence, becoming more similar in personality than they were in their younger years. This pattern appears to occur in numerous cultures. One explanation is that it represents a move toward "wholeness" of personality after the cultural and possibly biological emphasis on gender differences in behavior earlier in life, which has young men assuming the assertive roles and young women the nurturing ones.

People may also simply grow tired of their usual roles and desperately desire a change. Sexual boredom and apathy are very common among older couples, who may fall into routine patterns in which they do the same things time after time, year after year, with little imagination in technique or style and a scarcity of zest for creating sexual excitement. Eventually the couple may no longer even care for each other. A new partner may seem to bring improvement, but unless the sources of the underlying boredom are dealt with directly, the improvement may prove only temporary after the novelty has worn off.

Interestingly, relationships that were unstable and unsatisfactory earlier in life sometimes improve in the later years, as the children grow up and leave and the stresses of parenthood and career pass. Personality growth may even lead to greater compatibility. On the other hand, long-standing problems between partners can worsen as the result of chronic irritation from years of unresolved conflict. Personality and behavior changes may also be unilateral: one partner may begin to move in new directions, leaving the other one behind, often angry and hurt.

What should you do if you and your partner are having problems? First, talk to each other about the problems—often. It is important to determine the basis of the problem and then to attempt to resolve it jointly. This, of course, is easier said than done. Be prepared for

233

the fact that each of you may refuse to admit your own contribution to the situation and may place the blame on the other. It is difficult to be open and objective about emotional issues, but it is absolutely essential to realize that what you should be looking for is a *solution* rather than a *culprit*. If you find that you can't get anywhere in trying to talk, go together to your clergyperson, your physician, or a professional psychotherapist or counselor. If your partner won't go, go alone. Late-life separation and/or divorce can be extremely painful and jolting; make the effort to salvage and improve the difficult relationship first. Even if a separation finally occurs, you will be comforted by the notion that you tried, and you will have learned something about yourself and your partner that may help you understand the past and prepare for the future.

Divorce

Currently 40 percent or more of first marriages end in divorce. Of the divorced, 67 percent remarry within five years. Recent years indicate that we may have stabilized at the current rates of divorce for the present. Some believe that there will be a trend back to preservation of marriages through more skilled premarital and marital counseling (counseling now prevents divorce in only

10 to 15 percent of cases, and conciliations have even less success) and less accessible divorces. Others see the tendency toward remarriages—"serial" marriages—as natural and inevitable as people live longer, divorce is easier to obtain, and women are more independent financially.

This was the case with Patricia, who was finally ready to admit that she wanted a divorce. She had spent forty-five years married to a self-centered, demanding man. Her two sons were in their forties, married and established. Patricia felt she might have a chance to build a new life in her later years. Her husband Herbert was shocked. He couldn't imagine what was wrong. Yet Patricia's desperation and despair were obvious. The two of them were vastly incompatible in personality, interests, and goals. After an effort at marital counseling, they broke up. Herbert never fully understood what happened to his marriage, but he quickly found another partner and remarried. Patricia relished her new freedom and began to find her own place in the world.

The process of separation and divorce precipitates more couples into professional counseling than any other life crisis, simply because it is so common and so frequently painful. Studies show that, at younger ages, men tend to have greater psychological adjustment problems after divorce than women, although women have far more economic problems, especially if they have children to raise. In the older age groups, the current generation of women appear to have the greater adjustment problems: their financial situation is more precarious, many have no work history outside the home, there are fewer men available for companionship and possible remarriage, and socially, older women alone are often stereotyped as boring and uninteresting. Yet significant numbers of older, divorced women report that they have built interesting and even exciting new lives for themselves.

Separation and divorce can have serious effects on your belief in yourself as a socially and sexually desirable person—particularly if it was your partner who initiated the process. The challenge is to build relationships in which you find support, social approval, friendship, and possibly a new intimacy with another person. We have outlined some suggestions for doing so later in Chapter 9.

YOUNGER WOMEN/ OLDER MEN

Younger partners of older men frequently express concern about male potency as men reach their sixties. Sometimes the anxiety is unfounded and reassurance is all that is necessary. But there can be real problems and then the young woman's question is "Is there anything that I can do?" The answer is yes, much of which is reviewed in this book. But one point is especially worth emphasizing. Clyde Martin of the National Institute on Aging's Baltimore Longitudinal Study on Aging reports that the capacity of older men for erotic imagery appears somewhat reduced with age. Since so much of sexual desire and performance originates in the mind, this is an important finding. The couple should openly discuss the issue and experiment with increasing their erotic stimuli. What works will be different for each person, whether it involves romantic settings, dancing, erotic films, videos and magazines, music, massage, and the like. Women also need to remember that manual stimulation of their partner's penis is often not only desirable but also necessary after midlife. And finally, reassurance and thoughtfulness on the part of women go a long way in resolving difficulties that may occur as men grow older.

RETIREMENT

Retirement can bring problems as well as possibilities for enhancing relationships. The sudden onset of twenty-four hours a day of togetherness can be a difficult adjustment to make! Such unremitting intimacy places greater pressure on emotional relationships and brings problems into more acute focus, so that what may previously have been an occasional irritant becomes a constant one. A struggle for control over daily activities can become a preoccupation as each partner strives to adjust to the other's frequent presence. Even if you can work out these struggles, the constant togetherness may dismay, disconcert, or irritate you. You must find a balance between shared time and time alone to give each of you elbow room, and you must talk to your partner about your concerns. In the future it is likely that more people will stay in the work force longer, either out of economic necessity (to support longer lives) or personal preference. But eventually a slowing down or stopping of outside work becomes a reality for most people and "togetherness" arises as an issue.

Yet, retirement has many advantages. Couples have more time to devote to relationships, and many in fact become closer to each other and to other people after full or even partial retirement. Schedules are also much more flexible, so that one or both members of a couple are less likely to find themselves exhausted when the opportunity for lovemaking arises.

CHRONIC AND INCAPACITATING ILLNESS

Illness may incapacitate one sexual partner physically and/or mentally but not the other, particularly when there is a substantial age gap between them. Frequently the man develops a serious illness first, leaving the woman without a companion or a sexual partner. Healthy women—especially those who are significantly younger than their husbands—may thus spend years in a relationship without adult intimacy or sexual contact. Other feelings can further complicate the picture. When one partner becomes ill, the other ordinarily reacts with concern and the desire to help. But if the illness becomes chronic, the healthy partner may be surprised to find himself or herself filled with anger. This may reflect a defense against the possible loss of the other, but it can also represent overwork, exhaustion, and/or an understandable resentment over missing out on life because of the duties of the nursing role and the incapacities of one's partner.

A woman attorney wrote us:

I am a consultant to our local committee on aging and have been asked in private conferences with persons over sixty what the attitude of a spouse should be whose husband/wife is hopelessly ill with dementia in a nursing home. In these cases the future time element is entirely uncertain, but much of the time the patients receive such good care that they may live for years and years and years. Have you written anything on this? Or can you refer me to something that has been written from a realistic viewpoint? I am familiar, of course, with the "moralistic" church view that you are married for life. But this is cold comfort to the healthy spouse with a desire to live a full, stimulating, and satisfying life.

It is important that you do not feel guilty about resentments and a sense of burden in the caregiving role. Face your feelings frankly and secure outside help whenever possible from your relatives, neighbors, friends, or professional homemakers to reduce your burden. Support groups involving people in similar circumstances can be very helpful. You may recognize that it is necessary to build new friendships to provide a sense of self-worth and companionship.

At other times physical illness may cause sexual problems, but despite this, you and your partner may still desire and be able to have a relationship that involves closeness and a sense of being valued. A woman tells us that she and her partner are in their seventies. Of her partner she says, "He's never lost his love and tenderness. He's always been a good lover." Yes, they still make love. But they no longer have intercourse because he has prostate cancer.

Again, intercourse is the form of sexual activity that is most likely to be impaired. Both you and your partner may feel guilty, so reassure each other that you can express your sexuality in other satisfying ways. In general, the less goal oriented (in terms of erections and orgasms) and the more flexible you both are, the more likely you both are to develop ways to enjoy lovemaking and each other.

Those with ill or disabled mates at home state that it is difficult to routinely bathe, feed, and provide nursing care for a mate and still think of him or her as sexually desirable. If sexuality is viable and important to you as a couple and you can afford help, hire a visiting nurse or a home-help attendant to take care of the less aesthetic parts of patient care. Returning to your normal roles as quickly and closely as possible is the goal. Other ways to adapt positively to the change are to express your feelings to someone you trust, or possibly to your partner; this way you can gather accurate information about your partner's physical problems, become involved in whatever rehabilitation process is feasible, and, if necessary, learn to express caring and sexuality in new ways.

At times a sexual relationship becomes totally untenable. For example, Judy's memory had become increasingly obliterated during the course of Alzheimer's disease. She had always said that she wouldn't want to live if she couldn't have her independence. It had never occurred to her that she might lose her intellectual abilities, her memory, and even her capacity to recognize her loved ones. Her husband, Jim, remained faithful and loving and was her major caregiver. When he would try to feed and dress her, she often became hostile and would even strike out at him. Jim had long ago lost his sexual desire for her. When he was simply holding her affectionately, she often resisted him or would even push him away. At other times she seemed aroused and would press him sexually, and he found it difficult to respond. Jim found relief by joining a group of caregivers with similar problems. He quickly learned to accept his reactions without feeling guilty or disloyal to the memory of his long and mostly happy relationship.

As strange as it might seem, the knowledge that an illness of one partner may be terminal or fatal sometimes brings an improvement or a heightening of a relationship. Couples report that the certainty or closeness of death causes them to cherish the present and to take advantage of the time they have left together. When sexuality is a part of that closeness, such couples should always have the opportunity for privacy and time alone, even if one partner is confined to a hospital or another institution. If you encounter problems in working this out with an institution, discuss the situation with the administrator, a patient representative, or a social worker on staff.

INSTITUTIONAL LIVING

The 5 percent of persons over sixty-five who live in homes for the aging, nursing homes, chronic-disease hospitals, and other long-term-care institutions are in general denied the opportunity for any private social and sexual life. Visitors are often in full view of room-mates and staff and can easily be overheard by them. Even those who have marital partners are seldom able to share conjugal visits, as they usually are not afforded a private time and place with their partners.

As to unmarried people who reside in nursing homes, intimacies of any kind—even hugging, kissing, or holding hands—may be frowned on despite the fact that they are performed by consenting adults. Even those who understandably resort to self-stimulation because they have no other sexual outlet run the risk of being discovered and reprimanded like children. When dementias of various kinds render people unable to make responsible decisions about sexuality, the nursing home staff should be carefully trained and supervised to handle sexual activity with kindness, good judgment, and appropriate restraints that respect the rights and feelings of the older person and those affected by his or her actions.

Nursing home administrators are often the key to how residents' sexual expression is viewed and responded to by nursing home staff. The late Jacob Reingold, vice chair of the Hebrew Home for the Aged at Riverdale, in the Bronx, New York, is said to have created the first sexual policy and procedure for a long-term-care institution in the United States. Reingold's policy states: "The resident's rights respect the importance of emotional and physical intimacy. . . . Residents have the right to seek out and engage in sexual expression, including words, gestures, movements, or activities including reaching, pursuing, touching, which appear motivated by the desire for sexual gratification." However, in recognizing that sexual expression is not always appropriate, due to complicated reasons involving mental capacity as well as personality conflicts in a group living situation, Reingold added, "Expressions of intimacy should not infringe upon the rights and reasonable sensibilities of others in the Home community."

Most older persons living under less enlightened conditions than those just described are reluctant to complain to the management, even though their rights as adults are being seriously infringed. Ask the administrator of your particular institution to provide whatever privacy you and other residents should have. If you need outside support, ask your relatives, friends, doctor, lawyer, or a member of the clergy to help you in stating your case. Speak to others who have a similar complaint and make it a joint project. If this fails, alert groups that are interested in the problems of older persons, such as local chapters of the Gray Panthers, the Older Women's

League, AARP (formerly called the American Association of Retired Persons,) and the Alliance for Retired Americans (formerly the National Council of Senior Citizens.)

Federal regulations issued on June 1, 1978, provide some right to privacy, but only for married couples, and only in nursing homes that participate in federal Medicare and Medicaid programs. These regulations are not being uniformly enforced, but failure to observe them *is* ground for legal action. For detailed information, contact the Health Standards and Quality Bureau, Office of Standards and Certification, Health Care Financing Administration, 7500 Security Blvd., Baltimore, MD 21244, Phone: 410-786-3000.

For guidelines on how staff should be trained to deal appropriately with residents' sexual relations, feelings, and help with problems that interfere with sexual functioning, see "Management of an Older Adult's Sexuality" in *The Textbook of Gerontologic Nursing*, Mosby Publishing, 1996.

A free consumer education program called *Love & Life: A Healthy Approach to Sex for Older Adults*, sponsored by the National Council on the Aging (NCOA), is available for use in any setting that involves older people, including nursing homes, homes for the aged, senior centers, adult day care centers, and the like. The complete *Love & Life* kit includes brochures, training materials, a videotape, an evaluation form for each participant, and other aids for use by organizations and professionals who work with older adults. Contact the National Council on the Aging, 409 Third St., S.W., Suite 200, Washington, DC, 20024, Phone: 202-479-1200.

WIDOW- AND WIDOWERHOOD

Unfortunately, the possibility of being widowed increases with age. Losses and grieving are inevitable as we grow older, and need to be worked through and accepted, so that the survivor may resume a full life or shape a new and different one. Losing someone you have loved—partner, friend, child—usually means shock and then a long, slow journey through grief. Acute grief, with the attendant mental anguish and remorse, ordinarily lasts a month or two and then begins to lessen. In most cases, grief works itself out in six to eighteen months unless further loss, stress, or other factors complicate it. *Widow or widower-shock*, an exaggerated state that can follow the sudden and unexpected death of a partner, or occur when the surviving partner is ill-prepared to handle living alone, leaves the survivor unable to accept death and take up life again. To recover, he or she needs to be encouraged to grieve and should be assisted in building an active life once more. The open expression of feelings, including crying, is important for both men and women in resolving their grief. Sharing your sadness, anger, resentment, fear, and self-pity with someone else helps.

Such *grief work* also involves talking about your sexual feelings. A newly widowed woman says of her sexuality:

> My husband died eight months ago. I would like some information about what happens to widows like me. I am surprised to find that one of the things I miss the most is my sex life. I feel so empty and alone now.

People need to separate out their own identities from the commingling of identities that has occurred in close and long-term relationships. The feeling that "part of me died with him [her]" can then be replaced with the feeling that "I am a person in myself and I am still alive." A man may find himself temporarily impotent, a symptom we call widower's syndrome; this usually clears up if he is encouraged to grieve and find his way through the loss.

Anticipatory grief, during which a person undergoes an extended grief reaction prior to the expected death of the loved one—as happens in the course of a terminal illness—can soften the shock of death. Although such grieving may result in a closer relationship with the ill partner, there are instances when the grieving person may close himself or herself off, as though the partner were already dead. If this occurs, you need outside counseling to reestablish the relationship with the dying person.

After the death of a partner, the man or woman who has been widowed may find it hard to look ahead to a new partner without feelings of guilt or disloyalty. In *enshrinement*, the survivor keeps things just as they were when the loved one was alive and spends his or her energy revering the memory of the dead person. The survivor believes that to live fully is a betrayal of love or loyalty for the dead. This survival guilt and fear of infidelity leads to emotional stagnation and stands in the way of achieving new relationships. Once the period of mourning is over and the initial shock and grief have abated, *you owe it to yourself* to become realistic about your need to have a new life of your own. This means you should preserve your memories appropriately, without excessive dwelling in the past. Jim, who is eighty-one, described his complicated feelings:

> I took care of Flo through the awful time—the diagnosis of her cancer, the chemotherapy, the radiation; it was miserable. She could not eat; for that matter, I couldn't either. We would hold each other, but that was about all. After a while, I have to say that it was not very pleas-

ant even to touch her. It was awful. I felt guilty about that. After she died, I grieved for a long time. I didn't think that I would want to have anything to do with anybody.

But about three months ago I met Marjorie at a school function for my grandson. She was a widow, too. She had lost her husband even before Flo died. It was like starting all over again. I was like a schoolboy. It took me some nerve to ask her to have lunch, but we did. We have gotten together a lot—to movies and dinner and various places—and I have held her hand and kissed her. But I feel guilty and disloyal to Flo.

In a support group designed for newly widowed persons, Jim learned that what he had been going through was *widower's guilt,* a common reaction in which the memory of one's dead partner becomes a roadblock to taking up life again. Jim participated enthusiastically in the group, and as the weeks went by, he began to build new relationships, including a compatible one with Marjorie.

The usual cure for both widower's guilt and enshrinement is to take an active role in getting life moving again. This is an act of will and determination. It can happen *only* if the individual decides to make it happen. You should remove from sight the personal possessions of the deceased, and put away such obvious marriage symbols as the wedding ring. It is *not* a betrayal of a past marriage to accept the present and build a future.

If your grief and anger over a death continue unchanged for years, then there is something interfering with the natural healing process of time. Quite often it is unresolved negative feelings toward the dead person (as in an unhappy marriage) or a stubborn refusal to accept fate and take positive steps toward creating a new life. In these cases, seek professional counseling.

For those aged fifty-five or older, AARP has a Widowed Persons Service in some 240 locations nationwide. A volunteer who has gone through the same experience will talk to the newly widowed person about his or her feelings, and help with any problems (write to: AARP, 601 E Street, N.W., Washington, DC 20049).

Remember, it *is* possible to develop a new, exciting and fulfilling life for yourself even *after* the death of your partner. A seventy-six-year-old widow recently let us know that. She wrote:

> I find myself in love with a wonderful gentleman of eighty-three years whom I met about six weeks ago after two months of letter writing. (He saw an advertisement I placed in the *Jewish Monthly*, looking for someone to correspond with.)
>
> I recently felt the need to write a poem about how I felt. Here it is:

WIDOW'S LOVE IN SPRING

Love in the Spring,
Can't do any old thing,
Just thinking of my Love
All day long.
Waiting to see him and feel his
Arms around me,
Wanting his lips on mine,
So tender and sweet.
Oh, the life of a widow
So happy and free
All because of
Love in the Spring.

Chapter 9

❧

WIDOWED, SEPARATED, DIVORCED, OR SINGLE: FINDING NEW RELATIONSHIPS

THE DEMOGRAPHIC DILEMMA

As they grow older, many people find themselves without partners. This is especially true of women because of their longer life expectancies and lower rates of remarriage after widowhood. Until medical science and public health programs (such as those aimed at prevention of late-life illness, disability, and, for many men, early death) become more successful in equalizing the life expectancies of men and women, we have to adapt to the social consequences of greater numbers of women after age sixty. Women are *already* adapting in a number of ways: by challenging negative cultural stereotypes of them, both personally and institutionally through organizations such as the Older Women's League and the Gray Panthers; by learning to take the initiative in building friendships and a social life; and by redefining their own sexuality to include a wider range of options for satisfying intimacy and sexual release. Some are developing relationships with younger men. Others have relationships with married men who may be unable or unwilling to leave their marriages. Some sublimate their sexuality by developing an interest in absorbing activities that bring them companionship and accomplishment. Lesbian women are in a particularly advantageous position as they reach midlife and beyond, since partners who are their own age will have a similar life expectancy, and they move in a world that becomes increasingly female with each decade.

None of this, however, negates the necessity of searching for ways to increase the life expectancy of men as well as preserving their physical vigor and sexual functioning as they grow older. Fortunately, we are already seeing improvements. There has been a 60 percent drop in deaths from heart disease and stroke since 1950 for white males, followed by a decline for black males beginning in the early 1970s. More recently, there has been a drop in lung cancer death rates for white males.

Overall disability rates for the older population are also showing some signs of decline.

Yet the likelihood of losing your partner is a fact of late life that increases with time, even by one's fifties. In 1998 over 46 percent of all women sixty-five and over were widowed compared to 15 percent of men. Another 4 percent of men and 5 percent of women this age had never married, and 6 percent of men versus 7 percent of women were divorced. Obviously there are differences between the lifestyles of those who never married and who over the years have created a circle of friends and intimates that substitutes for an immediate family, and those who are abruptly separated from a spouse by death or divorce and now find themselves on their own for the first time in many years or possibly in their lives. Where the widowed person is deprived of the shared intimacies and interdependence of long marriage and the social patterns that go with being a couple, the single or long-divorced man or woman is accustomed to living on his or her own. Still, as one grows older, time and deaths among one's peers erode the circle of relatives and close friends regardless of marital status. This can lead to an increasing emptiness in the later years that needs to be filled with new relationships.

BUILDING A NEW
SOCIAL LIFE

You cannot depend on the healing power of time alone to ease grief or loss or to alleviate loneliness. New relationships will not simply happen. You will have to take an active part in putting your life together again. Molly, age seventy-eight, and her late husband, Frank, had discussed their feelings long before he died. They had agreed that life should go on after one of them died, and that the survivor should feel free to explore new relationships and build a new life. This is exactly what Molly did. She became attracted to Ben, but decided to take her time before getting heavily involved with anyone. She did not want to rush into anything; it was time for her to enjoy her new life of dating and exploration.

Harry was sixty-one when his wife died of breast cancer. He and his wife had known Sarah and her husband George when they were all newly married in their twenties. Eventually Sarah and George divorced and Sarah went on to develop a thriving career. Harry and Sarah reconnected at a cancer fund-raiser organized by Sarah. At first both of them thought they had little in common. But as they reminisced about old times they started to see each other with a fresh outlook. They began to get involved in activities together, exploring whether an old friendship could evolve into new possibilities.

WHERE DO YOU START?

Take the initiative. It is up to you to take charge of your life, to decide what you want and what you should do about it. This does not mean you must be searching for a possible partner. You may want no more than opportunities to meet people who are congenial and likely to share your own interests. One way to do this is to look for activities that support these interests. You will feel less tense and pressured if you are doing what you like to do. A sense of pleasure and purpose in what you are doing will encourage you to enjoy, learn, give of yourself, and make friends.

SOME PEOPLE WORRY ABOUT ETIQUETTE

Those of you who are described as the "young old" (in your sixties) or are still in your fifties grew up in times of less inhibition about initiating relationships. However, many people even slightly older are still bound by the customs they learned as youngsters. Many of these formalities make no sense today. Women used to be told it was improper to call a man. But if you are interested, you do *not* have to wait for invitations from a man; simply behave as you do when you want to get in touch with a friend. He has the option of accepting or refusing, just as you do when a man (or woman) calls you. If he accepts your invitation, a friendship or a relationship may develop or it may not—but you will have taken a perfectly appropriate and dignified initiative that allows you an *active* role in finding new friends and activities.

WHAT ACTIVITIES SHOULD YOU TRY?

A variety of activities are available to older, single people who want to develop a fuller social life. Among the best opportunities are those afforded through work. More and more older people are remaining in the workforce, either from necessity, or choice, or both. A growing number are training for new careers or even joining the workforce for the first time, especially women. If you do not have a job but are interested and able, consider the possibility of looking actively for part-time work, both for the rewards of being useful and for the opportunities it offers to meet new people under daily and less self-conscious circumstances.

Where you live will affect the number of choices you have for activities that will widen your social circle. Except in isolated rural communities there are more possibilities than you may realize. If you are politically minded, for example, you can volunteer to help at your local political club. Volunteer work for worthwhile causes, social service agencies, or nearby hospitals or schools may provide you with personal rewards at the same time that it brings you into contact with other people who share similar concerns. Those who like to be active and out-of-doors can seek out health clubs, hiking and biking clubs, wilderness, nature, and bird-watching groups.

If you can't find something that fits your particular taste, consider organizing it yourself. Any special interests can lead to social contacts. Musicians can start amateur chamber music groups, orchestras, or jazz, western, country, and ethnic music groups. Many towns and cities have amateur choirs, where an interest in singing is the only prerequisite. Painting, theater, handicraft, and folk art clubs are popular; if there is a Y in your community, you may find it is already sponsoring such activities. One midwestern woman started a sewing circle aimed specifically at men who wanted to learn how to quilt and do needlepoint. Organizing potluck dinners is a good way to cut costs and promote sociability. Cooking clubs are popular among both men and women. Woodworking and carpentry, wine making and tasting, investment clubs, Toastmasters clubs, chess clubs, and bridge and other card and game clubs can be comfortable ways to meet people.

If you live in a city or its suburbs, you have the advantage of a wider choice of activities. Senior centers (for older people who enjoy their own age group) and community centers (for all ages) offer recreational opportunities; there are now at least ten thousand senior centers and clubs in the United States, operated by churches, synagogues, social clubs, and nonprofit corporations. These centers offer shows, parties, music, beauty salons, handicrafts, trips, discussion groups, and a variety of other things to do at the same time you are encountering new people.

Religious activities are another important way of meeting people. Many churches and synagogues sponsor singles clubs, and some are beginning to expand these to fit the needs of people in the mid and later years. Talk to your local cleric about starting such a group if one does not exist in your locale. If you are the parent of a child or an adolescent, Parents without Partners clubs (1650 South Dixie Highway, Boca Raton, FL, 33432, Phone: 561-391-8833) can be a source of contacts and of help to you, both as a parent and as a single person.

If you live in a rural area or a small town, you are more likely to know everyone who might be available as a friend or a companion in your area, just as they, in turn, know you. For variety you may want to make and visit friends in neighboring communities and get to larger urban areas for activities whenever possible. Trips and vacations away from home can be a way of making new acquaintances. If you don't have a car, arrange to share rides with others if you can. Neighbors and friends may be willing to serve as a taxi for you, or you may be able to go by bus.

A small but growing number of older people have begun to live together in communal settings as a means of increasing their social contacts, cutting costs, and sharing housekeeping duties. Some house-sharing groups are made up only of older people, while others include people of all ages. Most of these are in large houses, although we have also heard of large apartments that are occupied communally and are free of the chores of caring for a house and yard.

AARP (national office at 601 E Street N.W., Washington, DC 20049) may have chapters in your area where meetings of many kinds take place. Look on the Internet, in your phone book, or if necessary, check with the national office to see if there is a chapter near you. The AARP alone has thirty-four million members, which provides for significant political advocacy and services (such as discount drugs, insurance coverage supplemental to Medicare, low-cost travel) as well as social opportunities. Widowed older people have been finding support and direction for their lives through the Widow to Widow program, which originated in Boston and is now being sponsored in other cities by the AARP.

The other major membership organization for older people, the National Council of Senior Citizens, as of January 1, 2001, had been subsumed under a newly created AFL-CIO organization called the Alliance for Retired Americans, 815 Sixteenth Street, N.W., Washington, DC 20006, Phone: 202-637-5000. Its membership includes 2.5 million retired union members and other older and retired people and its goal is to sponsor a wide range of activities that will benefit older citizens.

If you would like to combine opportunities for meeting people with social and political activism, the Gray Panthers (733 Fifteenth Street N.W., Suite 437, Washington, DC 20005, Phone: 800-280-5362), works vigorously on behalf of the older population as well as cross-generational issues. It includes younger as well as older people in its membership. The National Caucus on the Black Aged (1424 K Street N.W., Suite 500, Washington, DC 20005, Phone: 202-637-8400) focuses specifically on the issues and concerns of older African American people. The National Association for Hispanic Elderly or *Asociación Nacional por Personas Mayores*, 1452 West Temple Street, Suite 100, Los Angeles, CA 90026-1724, Phone: 213-487-1922, is a resource for older Hispanics.

Ocean cruises can be fun, and some people do meet partners this way, although the cruises generally attract more women than men and are expensive. If you have the money, are interested in where you are going, and like to travel, you can enjoy yourself and make friends on a cruise. Don't be afraid to ask the ship's purser for help in meeting others and seating you with compatible dining companions. Younger men who are attracted to older women may use cruises as a meeting place; be careful that they aren't interested chiefly in your money.

A more inexpensive way to travel sociably is to go on bus tours, some of which cover the entire United States and parts of Canada. You can get a ticket for use nationwide at reasonable rates. Take a friend, go by yourself or with a group, and be open to meeting new people along the way. Planes and trains typically offer discounts, some of them substantial, to those over sixty or sixty-five.

The travel industry is actively promoting travel for single people of all ages, with special seminars, tips for solo travelers, and tour packages. Club Med (800-258-2633), the Sierra Club trips (415-977-5500), Smithsonian Tours (1-800-258-5885 for overseas tours), and Lindblad Travel vacations (booked through travel agents) are popular with single people. Travel Companion Exchange (800-392-1256) uses computerized listings to help pair single people for all sorts of travel—not just to arrange companions but to avoid the penalty many hotels, tours, and cruises place on single travelers. Other singles travel services are listed on the Internet using the keywords "singles travel."

The Elderhostel program (11 Avenue de Lafayette, Boston, MA 02111, Phone: 877-426-8056) is a not-for-profit organization with twenty-five years of experience in providing interesting travel and educational experiences at reasonable costs for those fifty-five and older. These are short-term programs (one to four weeks long) that provide for a comfortable mix of couples and single participants, as well as special room arrangements for singles, roommates as requested, and the like. Elderhostel is remarkable for its diversity and quality of national and international travel and learning opportunities in over ninety countries. There are lectures, field trips, discussions, and social activities but no tests or assignments in classes.

Dance lessons are widely touted for older people, but be wary: the commercial ones can be greatly overpriced and sometimes fraudulent, offering "lifetime contracts" and noncancelable contracts. If you can't locate a reputable and reasonably priced place to learn, find friends who will teach you. If you are a good dancer, offer to teach someone else. Consider square dancing, folk dancing, and especially ballroom dance. For example, the Roseland Ballroom in New York City is available for ballroom dancing on Sunday afternoons and evenings (predominantly frequented by older persons). Friendships and romances can begin in such settings— Roseland has a plaque on its wall engraved with the names of married couples who first met there. Summer outdoor dance venues are also becoming popular. New York, for example, has outdoor folk dancing on summer weekends in Central Park, as well as swing dancing on summer evenings in the Lincoln Center courtyard.

High school, college, and other reunions offer men and women the chance to renew acquaintances with compatible people they knew earlier in life, who are now widowed or divorced themselves. So go to them! It is not uncommon for childhood sweethearts to meet again and even permanently reconnect after each has raised a family and been widowed or divorced. One recent California study of one thousand people who had reunited in later life with an old flame from earlier times found that a "first love the second time around" has a better than average chance of a happy relationship. Several Internet sites specialize in helping find old friends, schoolmates, and work colleagues. ThirdAge.com, recently acquired by MyFamily.com, offers information and advice to persons from their midforties, fifties, and beyond, whom they describe as "first-wave baby boomers." One specialty is helping people track down and link up with former sweethearts.

Another site, Bigfoot.com, has a free-access database of 35 million e-mail addresses everywhere in the world. Classmates.com has collected more than 11 million names of graduates of nearly 50,000 American and Canadian high schools and secondary schools abroad. Michael Schutzler, the company president, claims a million users who are fifty-five or older and a dozen more in their nineties. He states that getting in touch with former classmates is "inevitably a positive experience, whether it is purging old demons or reliving fond memories." He plans to add alumni from colleges and universities to the database in the future. Finally, if all else fails, you can log onto USSearch.com, which locates people through a huge number of sources, including court records, government documents, and professional society databases. This site charges a modest fee for a quick search and a slightly higher fee for a more extensive search conducted by staff researchers.

Family reunions and family contacts in general are another way to get in touch with people who may be seeking new relationships; there is a long and honorable tradition, for example, of widows and widowers who are in-laws developing close relationships that end in partnerships or marriages.

Commercial singles clubs and computer dating services are growing in popularity, especially for the young and middle-aged, but older people are using them as well. The Internet is becoming a common meeting place—but exercise caution. If you meet someone online and want to become acquainted face-to-face, arrange for initial meetings to take place in public spaces with lots of people around. You might also take a friend along. Keep all initial meetings in locations outside your home, preferably in settings where others whom you know can also get acquainted with the person and give you their feedback. Don't give out personal information unless you become comfortable that the person is legitimate and not exploitative or deceptive. And don't expect success too easily in finding someone interesting and suitable. As someone has wisely said, "You have to kiss just as many frogs on the Internet as through other methods." Among the ten top matchmaking Web sites ranked by the Nielsen/NetRatings are Personals@ Yahoo.com, Match.com, Relationships.com, and Friend finder.com. Smaller sites cater to specific interests, such as seniors, sports lovers, and the like. There is often a short-term free subscription, followed by an average fee of $20 a month to post personal profiles and respond to those of others. Browsing is usually free. If you need help navigating the matchmaking system, a site named XmeetsY.com may prove useful.

Next50.com is a fast-growing Web site that was begun in September 2000 and could become one of the largest on-line senior networks. It offers eighteen different information topics, including an elaborate "relationships" site that includes an advice columnist for those over fifty, a senior chat room, a search locale for finding an "activity partner" or a date, and access to licensed marriage, family, and sex therapists. It also offers Internet service provider (ISP) service designed for seniors.

The Internet is rapidly becoming a place for just plain sociability. A growing world of people meet regularly on-line to chat or to play checkers, bridge, bingo, backgammon, chess, and many other games, both old-fashioned and new. You can find a game and conversation twenty-four hours a day on dozens of sites. Men and women play in about equal numbers in all age groups. Pogo.com, bingo.com, and station.sony.com are a few of the popular game Web sites.

Personal ads, too, have become popular and even reputable. For a small fee you can dream up a description of yourself and the kind of partner you are looking for and place it in the classified section of a wide variety of newspapers and magazines. Your identity is protected by a post office box number unless and until you choose to reveal yourself to a respondent. As with Internet acquaintances, keep first meetings limited to safe, public locations.

If you are simply looking for an escort or temporary companion for a business or social event, there are legitimate agencies that will provide people, for a fee. Some escort services, however, are fronts for hiring sex partners (both male and female). If you are uneasy about commercial escort services, ask a friend or your local cleric whether he or she knows someone who could accompany you, or get in touch with an older persons' group or senior center.

Don't overlook born matchmakers among your friends, acquaintances, colleagues, children, or other family members. Some people have highly developed sensibilities and can be very helpful in finding men or women you would enjoy meeting. But save yourself time and trouble by picking your matchmaker carefully; look for someone whose judgment you respect and who knows you well.

QUALITIES THAT FOSTER NEW RELATIONSHIPS

When you first venture to meet new people, it will help to remember that they are as likely to be feeling as tentative, shy, or embarrassed as you are. And what you look for in other people—companionship, friendship, relationships—are usually the same types of things they are seeking from you. When you do strike up an acquaintance, be warm and sensitive to the other person's feelings. It doesn't matter if you are quiet or lively—everyone's temperament is different—but in either case, you'll fare better if you display curiosity and an active mind. People also appreciate imagination, responsiveness, and a sense of humor.

That said, there are certain personal qualities that foster the art of making friends. Most people respond to a sense of vitality and energy. Those who are pleasantly assertive (not domineering) have a greater chance of meeting new people and forming rewarding relationships—and it is simply because they do not leave all the initiative up to others.

QUALITIES THAT HINDER NEW RELATIONSHIPS

It is important to maintain a positive approach, one that transcends or tempers any problems you have. Many people have endured the deaths of spouses or friends, difficulties with children, financial burdens, loneliness, and an increasing feeling of uselessness. Under these pressures, it is not uncommon for you to feel that life has been unfair and to bear a grudge against your circumstances. But this resentment is likely to make other people wary of becoming involved with you. It is depressing to be with someone who is complaining or petulant and whose outlook is pessimistic. So make a deliberate, conscious act of will to overcome the perception that all seems sour in your life. If you don't do this, you'll be hindering your chances for new and enriching relationships.

CAN YOU BE EXPLOITED?

When someone "uses" someone else in an emotional relationship without giving much in return, it is exploitation. It is up to you—and only you!—to know what to look out for and how to protect yourself. Some older men (and, far more rarely, women) marry primarily to gain a housekeeper or nurse. Well, the "romance" is going to disappear as soon as the marriage vows are exchanged and the woman discovers she has been recruited primarily to perform these services. It is much wiser, of course, to take the time to learn as much as you can about the other person before you decide to marry. The history of his or her relationships with the opposite sex can be incredibly illuminating. Most exploiters have a long history of taking advantage of others.

In other instances the exploiter may primarily be after your money or property. Matrimonial swindles through lonely-hearts clubs and correspondence with strangers who claim a romantic interest in you are notorious. The tip-off comes when the person begins to be inordinately interested in your property, your money, or your will. *If you suspect this is happening to you, get to a lawyer, cleric, or someone else you can trust, and ask for advice.*

SPECIAL ISSUES FOR WOMEN

Unattached middle-aged and older women, especially those who are widowed or divorced, often find themselves left out of activities that involve couples. Hostesses at dinner parties feel they must have a man available for each woman guest, with couples coming two by two like the creatures on Noah's Ark. The hostess may also find the presence of a widow or divorcee uncomfortable because she fears possible competition.

If you are frequently left out socially, one solution is to join with other single people and organize your own activities. Or develop a circle of friends in which friendship rather than gender is the key to getting together, and where people of any age, sex, or marital status can enjoy one another's company. Start inviting your own married friends along; in the process they may become less inflexible about their own social habits in inviting guests!

If you are divorced, be prepared to have some people see you as a failure. They may make the conscious or unconscious assumption that the breakup of your marriage was caused by a flaw in you. This attitude is fast disappearing however, under the weight of demographic figures showing that half of all first marriages end in divorce. Get support by talking things over with under-standing and nonjudgmental people who care about you.

Both widows and divorcees find that some men (married or otherwise) assume that women who are sexually experienced are automatically available and willing. Indeed, these men may see themselves as doing you a sexual favor. If this expectation annoys or upsets you, tell them so. If they don't understand, write off the relationship.

Single women who have never married have their own set of concerns. Here is an example of someone with a relatively rare, special problem:

> Your book *Love and Sex after Sixty* is fine for married couples, but what about a single per-son who has never had sex? Naturally, I have always been curious, but I would be terrified to indulge. I never had a date until I was thirty, and every man I went on a date with expected sex in return. Out of fear, I stopped dating. Sex is for *after* marriage. Of course, I blame myself for not being married and you can't blame a man for trying. But the man who is looking for a wife doesn't want someone al-ready picked over, so I've remained single and lonely.

If this situation is yours, we recommend that you speak to a professional counselor who should be able to help allay many of your concerns. And there *are* men out there who are not looking for immediate sexual involvement.

SPECIAL ISSUES FOR MEN

As a general rule, unattached men have fewer *social* difficulties. Even those who had not thought themselves socially very accomplished when they were younger may be surprised to find how eagerly accepted and actively pursued they now are. (This is largely because there are fewer men than women.) One eighty-one-year-old man told us:

> I have scarcely had a moment alone since my wife died of a long illness last year. The ladies in my church have taken pity on me as "a helpless man," I guess. I had more food appearing at my front door than you could imagine—it was a regular casserole brigade for weeks after my wife died! I was in too much shock and upset at the time to see all the humor in this. But we men are in big demand in old age. I for one think it's great!

So if you are a man who enjoys relationships with women, you are likely to have ample opportunity for them! On the other hand, if you find it annoying or troubling to be treated like a commodity in short supply, you will have to make this clear or else remove yourself from those situations where this tends to occur.

Uncertainty can be a problem for men. Many men, like many women, are hesitant, shy, or dubious about their ability to handle personal relationships. To find yourself valued as an available man as you grow older is not automatically reassuring if you doubt your sophistication, skill, or appeal to the opposite sex. Most men have been conditioned to believe that anything short of total self-confidence is shameful, a failure of "masculinity." Though a woman may have similar problems of self-confidence, society has not pressured her into feeling "unwomanly" as a result. If you are troubled by doubts about your skill in social and sexual situations, recognize that you have plenty of company, and that this insecurity reflects in no way on your degree of manliness. Most women you meet are not going to measure you against some impossible ideal and judge you a failure. Further, the man who is shy, diffident, or uncertain about his competence will have to make the same effort of will, and exercise the same degree of initiative, that a hesitant woman must undertake. You will discover if you do not take this step that relationships are no more likely to happen for you than they would for her.

SPECIAL ISSUES IN LESBIAN, GAY, BISEXUAL, AND TRANSGENDER RELATIONSHIPS

It has long been a societal belief that life becomes increasingly bleak and lonely as the lesbian, gay, bisexual, or transgender (LGBT) person grows older. This is an outmoded and simplistic supposition that requires examination. An estimated 4 to 5 percent or even more of all Americans characterize themselves as LGBT (a relatively new term designed to include transgender persons—namely those who identify as the opposite of their original gender—in the larger lesbian and gay community); and, similar to the majority heterosexual population, many have long-term relationships, are emotionally stable, and as successful and happy (or the reverse) in their later years as other groups. (Note: individuals who identify as "transgender" may be heterosexual, homosexual, or bisexual—a fact that touches on the complexity of attempting to categorize such groupings.)

When difficulties, both social and sexual, occur for LGBT couples and individuals, they involve many of the same interpersonal problems faced in heterosexual relationships. But in addition, LGBT older persons may find themselves isolated in the larger society, with too few role models for growing older as members of a partnership or as single people. There can be a lack of support from friends, relatives, and others when a longtime

companion is ill or dies. Often hospitals and other institutions do not recognize the LGBT relationship in terms
of visitation rights and consultation with medical personnel. Legal rights are often unclear and unprotected;
for example, relatives of the deceased can and do contest
wills if belongings are left to the deceased's partner.

The current generation of LGBT elders grew up
in a difficult era of change and challenge. Before the
turn of the twentieth century, few nonheterosexuals in
the United States had any sense of community with others like themselves, or any feeling of acceptance in the
larger world. Most married and either lived double lives
or suppressed their sexual inclinations. Midcentury
brought greater freedom, especially for those in large urban areas. But it was not until the late 1960s, when the
modern gay liberation movement began, that the LGBT
community forged a real sense of solidarity and won
greater social acceptance. Thus, many older individuals
have gone through major struggles both personally and
socially. A good number are still in the closet, living as
"roommates," "sisters," "brothers," and so on. Many
also face the tremendously complicated challenge of the
AIDS crisis, which has drawn both attention and resources away from other issues of aging in the gay community (see the section on AIDS on pages 93–101).

Nonetheless, organizations *are* beginning to form to
aid LGBT individuals as they reach their later years.
SAGE (Senior Action in the Gay Environment) at 208
West 13th Street, New York, NY 10011, Phone: 212-

721-2247, offers a variety of social services to older members in the New York metropolitan area and promotes the opportunity for intergenerational support. In 1992, SAGE developed SAGE-NET, a group of independent affiliates in the United States and Canada that share SAGE's mission. Contact them for their newsletter, *SAGE News & Events.*

The Lesbian and Gay Aging Issues Network (LGAIN), sponsored by the American Society on Aging (833 Market Street, Suite 511, San Francisco, CA 94103, Phone: 415-974-9600), is a professionally-oriented umbrella organization providing links to other LGBT organizations, researchers, and publications. LGAIN publishes a quarterly newsletter, *OutWord,* which offers a comprehensive, ongoing source of information about LGBT aging.

The National Association of Lesbian and Gay Gerontologists is actively promoting understanding and service for the LGBT community in mid and later life. It offers a quarterly newsletter, *Making a Difference,* and has compiled *Resource Guide: Lesbian and Gay Aging*; both can be obtained by writing to The National Association of Lesbian and Gay Gerontologists, 1853 Market Street, San Francisco, CA 94103.

New Leaf Outreach to Elders (formerly known as GLOE—Gay and Lesbian Outreach to Elders), 1853 Market Street, San Francisco, CA 94103, Phone: 415-255-2937 or 415-626-7000, offers a monthly newsletter, *Outreach to Elders,* and provides services to lesbians, gays, bisexuals, and transgender persons sixty years and older. New Leaf offers information, referral, counseling, support groups, social activities, friendly visiting for elders, trips, a legal clinic, education forums, and special events.

Lesbian women may wish to write for *Golden Threads*, P.O. Box 1688, Demorest, GA 30535-1688, a publication for lesbians over fifty and those involved with them, with the purpose of making it possible, in a caring and confidential way, for lesbians to develop friendships even when they are socially or geographically isolated. This quarterly publication has an international circulation and contains editorials and book reviews slanted toward the interests of older lesbians; it also includes a large resource list.

Dignity/USA Task Force on Aging (a Catholic lay organization), at 1500 Massachusetts Ave. N.W., #11, Washington, DC 20005-1894, Phone: 800-877-8797, developed guidelines for its local chapters on the subject of older lesbians and gay men. It published a nationwide directory of organizations/services for older lesbians/gay men and developed a resource packet for workshops.

For legal guidance, *The Legal Guide for Lesbian and Gay Couples*, 10th Edition, by Hayden Curry, Editor (Nolo Press, 1999) covers important legal and financial aspects of lesbian and gay relationships.

It is important to note that research in the LGBT community is moving toward greater fine-tuning in order to draw attention to more specific aspects of LGBT life, including aging processes. Examples are research directed at the gay male or lesbian couple aging together; bisexual and transgender aging couples; the "gay widow"; the single older gay, lesbian, bisexual, or transgender person; aged gay men and lesbians in the larger gay community; special therapy and counseling needs of the older LGBT person; and adult children of older LGBT couples. Please also refer to the bibliography at the end of this book, which lists a number of titles of special interest to the LGBT community.

AS A RELATIONSHIP DEVELOPS

New anxieties may occur as a relationship progresses to sexual involvement. When men or women doubt their sexual performance, or fear that the person with whom they are involved may be measuring them against the behavior of a previous partner, it will affect their sexual ability. It takes an active effort by both you and your current partner to make the present moment satisfying. Do not allow memories of past lovemaking to dominate the present. What each of you can give the other should concern you more than anything else, and especially more than anything that was in the past. If a caring person offers reassurance to a partner who is feeling uncertain about his or her skill, it will help restore confidence. Yes, deeply rooted sexual problems may require professional help, but the self-doubt that has its roots in shyness and uneasiness about performance—which is much more common—is often alleviated by thoughtfulness and tenderness.

HANDLING REFUSALS, REBUFFS, AND DISAPPOINTMENTS

However confident they may appear on the surface, a great many men and women worry about rebuffs when they initiate or respond to a social opportunity. How can you best handle such refusals and disappointments? It *is* natural to feel hurt, but you should not let this feeling persist. You have to face the possibility of rejection whenever you involve yourself with others, so be matter-of-fact about it. It is, after all, the other person's right— as it is yours when you are approached. It should not deter you from further involvements. Remember that *rejection is nature's way of keeping two people apart who should not be together.* Trust that there is someone out there who will suit you better.

Obviously, there will be some occasions when a person rudely rejects you and doesn't take into account your feelings. These times will be unpleasant and sometimes painful. This is an unavoidable aspect of human relationships. The point to remember is that *refusals or disappointment do not mean you are a failure as a person.* If you are losing confidence and feel you need a fresh perspective on yourself, talk over your experiences with a close friend. Then draw on the experience you have gained and try again. Take a few chances. Above all, do not waste time berating yourself for what does not work out. Not everything is your responsibility; some aspects of relationships are out of your control.

MOVING TOO FAST

What if one partner in a newly acquainted couple moves too quickly toward intimacy? There is always the widow who is husband-hunting or the man who is on the make sexually on the first date. Carla, age sixty, had met the latter:

> I liked Max immediately when I first met him. (He's sixty-four.) But he was too fast for me: He just barged ahead without looking for any signals. He seemed hell-bent on sex. Now that I think about it, he has had three marriages and two of them have been divorces. He probably has made a habit of demanding his own way. Maybe I'll tell him what I think. What have I got to lose?

Use your common sense and don't be afraid to tell the other person if you are feeling pushed. You have the right to have your feelings respected. If you are one of those impulsive or action-oriented individuals, be sensitive to your companion's feelings. A relationship that is going to be more than merely temporary needs time to build. Explore each other's feelings and learn more about each other. Decide *together* what pace to set. Many people are not ready for physical intimacies—much less marriage—until they feel a mutual understanding and affection. An enduring partnership is based on thoughtfulness as well as attraction. If he or she is not willing to provide you with the time that you need, it may simply mean that there is someone else out there more suited to your temperament.

ARRANGING FOR PRIVACY WHEN YOU LIVE WITH YOUR CHILDREN

Living with your adult children or having them live with you—as roughly 20 percent of older people do—can certainly put a damper on your social life unless you take preventive steps. And don't depend on your children to recognize your needs for privacy. You will need to take the initiative and discuss this with them frankly. Work out ways of sharing the space in the home, so that there will be times when you can entertain people privately. Some houses are large enough for you to have your own suite of rooms, which makes a separate social life easier. But most older people who live with relatives will have a bedroom at most, and sometimes even this will have to be shared with another member of the family. If you have your own room and it is a reasonable size, you can furnish it as a combination bedroom/sitting room and entertain your friends there. If small children live in the house, put a lock or latch on the door to keep them from running in and out until they learn to knock and enter only on invitation. Your bed can be a couch by day, and you should also have a comfortable chair and other amenities for entertaining. If you must share a bedroom, arrange to have sole use of the room at certain times. There may be difficulties in entertaining privately in the family living or dining room unless you and your family have worked out a practical schedule. It is easier if there is also a recreation room or den. If your resources permit, finance the construction of additional space or undertake some remodeling to gain desired privacy.

It is extremely important that you make your children aware of your desire for privacy *before* you move in with them or they with you. Discussing the issue before actual situations arise is more likely to produce results. When they are moving in with you, things are usually a bit easier because you are on your own territory. The crucial element in living successfully with your children in their home is to be able to talk openly with them about problems and cooperate in solving them.

UNMARRIED AND LIVING TOGETHER

Many couples who come to care for each other want to marry; for them marriage confirms the permanence and depth of their commitment. In addition, for some older people the idea of living together without marriage goes against their moral or religious scruples. But the number of unmarried men and women of all ages living together as sexual partners has increased from two million in 1984 to nearly three million in 1990. Little is known about the myriad reasons unmarried older persons live together. The decision a couple makes may involve deliberate choice, but it also may be the result of necessity. Two people may care deeply for each other but feel that marriage would set limits on an independence they have come to value. Many older men and women who nursed partners through a long chronic illness until death may now feel they do not want to enter into another marriage that might put them through that same ordeal all over again.

There are also instances in which marriage is not an option, and people embark on affairs. Everyone knows of unhappy marriages that continue for years because one partner will not agree to divorce, in effect forcing the other to seek a partner outside marriage. In other marriages, one member may have been incapacitated or chronically ill for a long time, leaving the other without a satisfying sexual and emotional outlet. Affairs are more likely to occur if the marital couple had an unsatisfying emotional relationship to begin with, or if one partner is mentally impaired or institutionalized.

Sometimes the children of a widowed parent object strongly to his or her dating or remarrying. This may cause the parent to avoid relationships because of the fear of family conflict. If this happens, you owe it to yourself to initiate discussions with your children to resolve your differences. If all else fails, call in an outside objective mediator.

Economic factors may also enter into decisions not to remarry. While recent legislation has improved this situation, there may be pension penalties in cases of remarriage. State Medicaid benefits can also be a barrier. If one partner has been receiving Medicaid, marriage would mean suspending that support until at least a major portion of the savings of the new spouse was used up; only then could Medicaid be resumed. Indeed, there have been cases where husband and wife divorced each other, but continued to live together in order for one of them to be eligible for Medicaid.

In general, the decision of whether to marry or to live together is a private one, to be reached by each individual couple. A host of influences can impact their decision, including religious attitudes, the reactions of relatives, financial considerations, and personal preferences. Everyone should go with the solution that best suits his or her individual circumstances.

CHAPTER 10

❧❧❧

LEARNING NEW PATTERNS OF LOVEMAKING

If you have been thinking about some aspects of your sexual life that you would like to change, *now* is the time to do it. Don't believe people who tell you that as you grow older you become too fixed in your ways to change. If you were always interested in learning and changing in your past, that attitude is likely to remain with you all your life. Besides, scientific studies have proved beyond question that older people can learn as well as, and in some cases better than, the young.

Nevertheless, be careful not to underestimate the strength of habit, which can be even greater when it is unconscious; lovemaking patterns tend to become fixed and uninspired over the years, often because you have neither taken the time nor thought it necessary to examine them. Well, it is now time to look with a critical eye at how you have been handling sexual intimacy. Do you always make love at the same time of day and in the same manner? Are you excited and interested in your love life? Do you and your partner know how to please each other? It may be time to loosen up and try something new. Learn to relish once again the special warmth and intimacy that are possible through love and sex.

THE SETTING FOR SEX

Look at your bedroom with a critical eye. Is it comfortable and pleasant? Is it a good place for sex? A firm, comfortable bed for two should be standard equipment unless illness, sleeping problems, or personal preference lead you to choose single beds. In this case the best arrangement is one double bed for making love, talking, and so on, with a single bed in the same room or another room when you are ready to separate for sleep. A double bed encourages the closeness and sharing that enrich a couple's sense of togetherness.

Many older people with health problems develop the habit of lining up their medications on their bed stands. This is both aesthetically unattractive and dangerous. When you are drowsy you may fail to read the labels, take the wrong pills in the middle of the night, or accidentally take too many. So place all medications out of sight, at a walking distance from the bed unless they are absolutely essential for emergencies (for example, nitroglycerin for those with heart problems). In addition to protecting yourself, you will not be continually confronting yourself and your partner with reminders of your pains or infirmities.

Another thing that has struck us about many older people's bedrooms is the gallery of family pictures—children, grandchildren, nephews, nieces, and ancestors—that often lines the walls. This is fine for a couple married for many years who feels comfortable in this setting, but it can be quite unnerving, to say the least, for a new partner who settles down expectantly in the bed only to find your relatives looking down on the proceedings. Be sensitive to your new partner's feelings. If family pictures are interfering with your love life, banish them to another room.

THE TIME FOR SEX

Finding the best time for sexual activity can greatly enhance a sexual relationship. Having sex exclusively at bedtime is an easy habit to get into over the years, especially if daytime privacy is hard to come by and the pressures of work and family crowd your days. Yet, this may not really be your favorite time, and if you are over sixty (or even younger), it may not be your most ener-getic period either. For those who are overstressed, over-worked, and want or need to make love at night, set aside several evenings a week, relax, and go to bed early, be-fore exhaustion sets in. As to other favorable times for lovemaking: Some couples sleep first and make love in the morning. Others wake each other in the middle of the night, when both have had some rest. Many men re-port greater sexual potency after a good night's sleep. The morning is a favorite time for many older people because they are rested and relaxed. Daytime naps when possible can make for greater vigor in the evening for those who prefer nighttime lovemaking by choice rather than by default. Experimenting with new times on week-ends, holidays, and vacations can be invigorating. When vacations away from home are not possible, take a vaca-tion at home. If you have the house to yourself, unplug the phone and let the outside world know you're not available. Then settle down and enjoy yourself.

Relaxation is quite conducive for putting you in the mood for romance. A warm bath or shower before sex can help, as can exchanging massages with your partner, turning the lights low, and listening to music. (Massage courses for couples are now available in many major cities as part of adult education programs.) A *small* glass of an alcoholic beverage can be a tension reliever—we recommend dry white wine or warm Japanese sake. Warm milk, while it may not be the world's sexiest drink, can be soothing as well.

WHAT YOU CAN DO FOR YOUR PARTNER

You can acquire an extensive technical knowledge about how to make love from books, tapes, lectures, and courses. (We've included some of the books on sexual technique in the bibliography.) In our opinion, however, the *technique* of sex has been overpromoted, making lovemaking seem more like a gymnastic workout than an expression of love. Naturally, you can learn much that is valuable, but always remember that skill and technique can *never* substitute for genuine warmth and affection.

What we do want to do is direct your attention to information that is especially relevant to older people. For older women, the most common sexual problem is the inability to achieve orgasm. *Frigidity* is the word often used to describe this situation, but it is an unfortunate term because it implies coldness and sexual indifference. This does not adequately or appropriately explain what happens to many women. Women who ordinarily are able to have orgasms will have times when they are unresponsive (luckily such times are usually short-lived), and their temporary loss of response can have many causes, among them tiredness, emotional upset, boredom, vaginal infections or other physical ailments, drugs, and lack of adequate stimulation of the clitoris. Also, the loss of estrogen during menopause can affect a woman's sexual response. In addition, numbers of women never attain orgasm through intercourse but can reach it through other means, such as stroking by their partner or through self-stimulation. Orgasm by any of these means is enjoyable. Others never manage to reach orgasm through any method, including masturbation. Their total lack of sexual response is ongoing, and can usually be traced to emotional attitudes that developed during the early years of life. For some women this condition is extremely troubling; for others mildly so; and the remainder do not consider it to be a problem at all. For those who desire to change this situation, it may be possible to do so, even at a later point in life. What can make the difference? A helpful and thoughtful partner, and/or professional counseling or sex therapy.

As for pleasing your partner, there is growing evidence that women may have a different view of sexuality from men, with women placing less importance on the act of sexual intercourse itself and more on the affection, cuddling, physical holding, talking, and sharing that may surround a sexual relationship. While there's no indication that women are less interested than men in achieving orgasm and sexual release, many women prefer sexual activities other than, or in addition to, intercourse. Female anatomy plays an important role in women's attitudes. The majority of women receive their primary sexual satisfaction from clitoral stimulation, and for them, direct or indirect clitoral stimulation is the initial requirement in producing female orgasm. Because of this, sexual intercourse is often not satisfying unless it involves direct manual stimulation of the clitoris. (A number of studies indicate that substantially fewer women achieve orgasm regularly through sexual intercourse than through other methods.) Men can learn to stimulate the clitoral area, whether by hand, by mouth, or by the penis itself, and women should tell them what is pleasurable and what is not. Finally, many older women have problems of lubrication and may require longer periods of sex play before lubrication actually begins. KY Jelly or other water-based lubricants can be used in the vagina if lubrication is insufficient.

Women can and should learn to be sensitive and helpful when men are having problems with potency. Try a new coital position by bending your knees and placing a pillow under your hips to elevate your pelvis, in order to more easily accommodate your partner's partially erect penis. Remember that touching the penis can stimulate erection, so learn to massage it. Do not pull it up toward the abdomen, where it will lose blood. Instead, push down, with pressure at the base of the penis, which will put pressure on major blood vessels to hold the blood that the penis already contains.

A woman can further the strength of an erection by literally stuffing the partially erect penis into her vagina and flexing her vaginal muscles until it achieves full erection. Many women like to hold the penis in their vagina after lovemaking. If they have developed their vaginal muscles, this may be possible even if the penis begins to become limp, as happens more quickly after orgasm as men grow older. Finally, we want to stress again that a woman need not feel obligated to "give a man an orgasm" every time they make love. Leave this up to the man to decide and concentrate on mutually enjoying the physical and emotional contact, as well as your own orgasm if it occurs.

Men and women can learn to accommodate each other's needs in other ways. If one of you is obese or has a protruding abdomen, for example, you will need to experiment to find a sexual position that allows the penis to reach the vagina. One accessible position is for the man to lie on his back while the woman sits astride him.

Today older people experiment more with various sexual positions, just as do the young. There are many alternatives to the standard missionary position of the woman underneath, on her back, and the man on top. The most common ones to consider are lying side by side, the woman on top, or the man entering the woman from the rear.

As we have indicated, there are also a number of satisfying sexual alternatives to intercourse. These include mutual stimulation of each other's genitals by hand as well as stimulation of other erotic areas of the body—the mouth, neck, ears, breasts, and buttocks. Some couples use these techniques as foreplay before intercourse. Others use them as substitutes, either because intercourse is not possible or because they prefer them.

Sex gadgets are generally a waste of money except for battery-driven vibrators, which many people find stimulating, and certain prosthetic devices, which can help a man maintain a rigid penis or which can substitute completely for one. Older women should avoid douching after sex with perfumed douches or using vaginal sprays. They are unnecessary and can cause infections.

SOLO SEX

Self-stimulation, or masturbation, is a common and healthy practice that usually begins in childhood. It is natural for all children to explore their bodies, and most children stimulate themselves sexually unless they are prevented by adults from doing so. There is evidence that self-stimulation is an important preliminary to adult sexuality, enabling people to learn to recognize and satisfy their sexual feelings. The *1999 Merck Manual*, a highly reputable source of medical information, reports that approximately 97 percent of males and 80 percent of females have masturbated at some point in their lives. The evidence seems clear that, although masturbation was once seen as a perversion and a cause of mental and physical disease, it is now recognized as a normal sexual activity that one can engage in throughout one's life.

Self-stimulation provides a sexual outlet for people—unmarried, widowed, or divorced—who do not have partners, as well as for husbands or wives whose partners are ill or away. Some people practice self-stimulation in addition to sexual intercourse, particularly if they prefer sex more frequently than their partner does or enjoy the variety masturbation affords. And as described earlier, many women experience more intense and more frequent orgasms through self-masturbation or mutual masturbation with their partners than during intercourse. Masturbation can continue until very late in life and has been reported by some people in their nineties. A 1983 Consumers Union survey found that 66 percent of men and 47 percent of women in their fifties masturbate with some regularity; over the age of seventy, 43 percent of men and 33 percent of women still masturbate. In fact, some people begin to masturbate for the first time after they grow older, particularly if they have no partner or become too physically incapacitated for intercourse.

Total abstinence from sexual activity over a period of time can be tension producing and may result in potency problems in men and loss of lubrication as well as vaginal shape in women. So it can be beneficial to free yourself from the notion that self-stimulation is unhealthy, immoral, or immature. A source of pleasure to be learned and enjoyed for its own sake, masturbation also resolves sexual tensions, keeps sexual desire alive, is good physical exercise, and helps to preserve sexual functioning in both men and women who have no other outlets. Vibrators can be useful aids in masturbation. Many people engage in sexual fantasies, which add to the pleasure of self-stimulation.

COMMUNICATING WITH YOUR PARTNER ABOUT SEX

It is often extremely helpful to talk with your partner about your sexual feelings. Many couples assume at first that they don't have to talk, since sex "comes naturally," but this is simply not accurate. Because people are all different, with unique likes and dislikes, it is naïve to assume that our partners can read our minds or know intuitively how to please us. Furthermore, it is often said that sex begins in the brain, by the stimulation of the imagination and by memory of previous sexual experience. Our mind may well be our most sensitive and reliable organ of sensuality, so you should exercise it.

Begin by discussing your feelings about sex. It may seem embarrassing or awkward at first, but it is usually worth it to continue. Then tell your partner what gives you pleasure and have him or her do likewise. Finally, try in every way possible to do what is pleasurable for each other. You may be surprised at what you don't know about your partner and what you may have been reluctant to admit about yourself. You can also reminisce, talking about your first memories of sex, your early sexual attitudes and those of your family, and perhaps your feelings about what it means to be a man or a woman. Compare notes on what you would most like to change about yourself and your partner sexually. However, do be thoughtful and kind about the way you express any dissatisfactions you may feel.

Some couples go so far as to share their sexual fantasies with each other. Such fantasies, which are part of most people's sex lives, involve any visual and sexually stimulating images one conjures up. Some people are excited by imagining forbidden or unavailable sex partners, settings, or practices. Others bring to mind sexual experiences from the past that have been especially exciting. Some couples even make up fantasies for each other. The use of sexual videotapes at home may enhance fantasy and sexual stimulation.

The value of fantasy is that it adds a new dimension to one's sex life. People who may be otherwise fond of their partners but not easily aroused by them as the years go by report that fantasies, including fantasies of their partners and themselves when they were younger ("fantasy reruns"), can often get things started and help in reaching orgasms. Use fantasy to override a physical disability or distract yourself from anxiety or other preoccupations. Mental imaging can be especially useful for those whose vision is impaired. Since poor vision can interfere with the vital transfer of visual stimuli into sexual arousal, fantasy may provide the means for recapturing those stimuli.

So far we have few useful studies about fantasy in mid and later life. It would be interesting, for example, to know whether people usually fantasize themselves and others as younger than their actual ages.

Peruse books on sexuality and emotional relationships to learn more about yourself and each other. It is useful and stimulating to take a fresh look from time to time at what you know about sexuality and at the current attitudes of society toward sex. We have recommended a number of books in the bibliography. (There are many more, but most of them assume a young and middle-aged readership.) There are now films and tapes specifically addressed to medical and other aspects of sexuality in the mid and later years that are available to both health-care professionals and the public. Seek these out as well.

CHAPTER 11

❧❧

DATING, REMARRIAGE, AND YOUR CHILDREN

Many conflicts develop between parents and their adult children when a widowed or divorced parent attempts to build a new life through dating and, possibly, remarriage. To wit: "My daughter doesn't like my fiancée and thinks she is only interested in my money." "My son Jim feels I'd be a fool to marry Harry, since Harry has always been a ladies' man." "My children think I'm crazy to want a man. I wouldn't dare tell them what I did on my cruise to Jamaica."

Not all children create such problems. Many are pleased and, indeed, relieved at the thought of their parents leading full and satisfying lives. Others have realistic worries about the practical implications of these new lifestyles; they may welcome the remarriage of a father to a somewhat younger woman, because she will be able to nurse him as he grows older, but may feel threatened if their mother marries an older man, because it will be a burden on her, and potentially on them if he should fall ill.

For still other children the reactions are entirely emotional. The thought of a parent becoming involved with a new partner can provoke such strong emotions as anxiety, jealousy, hurt, fear, anger, or grief. In response they may be strongly inclined to offer unasked-for advice and even to "take over" if they feel a parent is making a mistake. Resorting to coercion, threats, and angry withdrawal are not at all uncommon.

As to why adult children react so negatively, there are numerous reasons. Those who never became fully independent psychologically use their parents to fulfill emotional needs that should be met by their partners and friends. You can assume this is the case if your child acts possessive or personally aggrieved, not unlike a wounded lover, when you become involved in a relationship. It is possible that you yourself (perhaps unconsciously) have encouraged an inappropriately close relationship with this child, or that other circumstances have kept the child from emancipating him- or herself. Age does not factor into these situations. Your fifty-year-old child can be dependent in this way even though he or she is married and has children. Under these circumstances, the best approach is to let your children know, kindly but definitely, that you intend to lead your own life, and to encourage them to do likewise.

Sometimes you may find that your children cling to the parental image of you as Mom or Dad and do not recognize (or want to recognize) that you need love and sex just as they do. Probably you have encouraged this attitude yourself by playing only the parent role whenever you were around them. A good antidote is to tell them more about your social interests and to bring your friends and dates home to meet them. You can still retain your privacy, but they should become aware that you are entitled to emotional and personal commitments. Though they may never feel entirely at ease about your right to a sexually satisfying life, they can often be helped to come to terms with its reality.

Children will sometimes try to preserve the memory of their deceased parent (or of your former relationship with a divorced spouse) by the process of *enshrinement*, discussed earlier in terms of widowhood. They maintain a fierce reverence for the past and want to see nothing changed, so they consider any new relationships you enter into an affront to their other parent. They may then accuse you of being selfish, insensitive, or disloyal; and if they succeed in making you feel guilty, you may be compelled to sever your new relationship. *This is a mistake.* Your children need to work through their own anger and grief at the death (or divorce) that ended your marriage. They are often bound to the past by a mixture of positive and negative feelings, and it is this ambivalence that must be resolved. Talk to them about their feelings, listen to their reactions, and try honestly to answer questions and clarify confusion. Also, let them know how you have handled your own feelings about their other parent.

Another problem can develop if your children have grievances or hold grudges against you, which they demonstrate by refusing to condone your right to build a new life for yourself. Some of these grievances may be lifelong, others recent; some may be misconceptions and misunderstandings of your actions toward them (particularly during their childhood), and others may be legitimate. Adult children easily become critical of their parents if their parents were always critical of them. Others remember being harshly punished or humiliated for innocent sexual experiences in childhood and have grown up thinking sex is wrong or dirty—and this might now include the sex lives of their parents. If you can begin listening openly to their grievances—even though it may be difficult—there is a chance that you and your children can develop a new understanding and respect for each other. Be ready to admit where you may have failed, but don't take the blame for everything. Your children and your former partner played their roles, too. The point is not to pin down a culprit, find a "bad guy," or allay grievances by making yourself a martyr, but to clarify what happened, why it happened, and whether anything can now be done to build a better relationship. Frank talk itself sometimes heals old wounds. And when it doesn't, *you* decide what choice you are going to make.

Next, we must look at a problem that can terrorize

a parent—the spoiled child. This is the child who grows up believing he or she is inordinately important and never stops believing it. Every spoiled child has one and usually two parents who were easily intimidated, over-indulgent, or lax with discipline. A favorite tactic of such a child is to threaten to withdraw love if the parent does not cater to his or her wishes. This tactic is all the more devastating when the child grows to middle age and attains greater power as the parent becomes older and loses status and authority. The sooner you get a hold on this situation, the better. *Do not let your son or daughter dictate to you.* It isn't good for you, and it certainly isn't good for your child. It may be frightening to think of losing this love, but remember that children rarely "divorce" their parents (if they do so, it is usually for a limited period of time, to try to get their own way), particularly if they know that basically you care about them.

Spoiled children have an intuitive understanding of power; they learned to use it expertly at a very early age. Use power in your turn to let them know the score. First of all, *keep your grip on your own money and property.* Then make your own decisions, particularly about your personal life. Get outside authority figures to help you if you need them in the initial battles that are bound to come. Your lawyer, your cleric, or a respected friend or family member may be able to support you when you waver, or speak for you if at first you can't. Be heartened by the knowledge that spoiled children usually develop respect for people who refuse to be manipulated.

Finally, we come to a most painful problem: the child who has one eye on your will. He or she is found particularly in those families where there will be a sizable estate after a parent's death. This child is forever worrying about his or her share of your estate and casts a cold eye on anyone you may be dating or thinking of marrying. Such a child will often plant suspicions in your mind that any close friend or prospective mate is after whatever money you have. Unfortunately, this happened to an attractive and vigorous widow we knew named Margaret. She had known Nathan only a short time and was surprised at how happy she felt when she realized that he was in the same room, or when his name was mentioned. She hadn't felt that way since her husband's courtship during their youth. Nathan and Margaret began to date and, eventually, to talk of marriage. However, to Nathan's astonishment, as soon as the talk turned to marriage, his children became extremely negative toward Margaret. They told their father that they were sure that she was a gold digger. He was horrified, but he had always trusted his children's opinions and so decided to hold off on marriage for a while. In turn, Margaret was justifiably hurt, and Nathan's decision changed their relationship. She felt wrongfully accused. Nevertheless, Nathan could not proceed wholeheartedly without his children's acceptance. The impasse finally gave way to alienation, and Nathan and Margaret sadly went their separate ways.

Don't let this happen to you. While older people

can be and have been exploited, if your mind is sound, you should rely on your own judgment and perhaps that of trusted friends or advisers—*not* on a child with a reputation for an obsessive focus on money or an inclination to avarice. (If you begin to have any questions about your own judgment, you can seek legal advice to set up a conservatorship. This will protect you, your funds, and your estate.)

What makes a child obsessive about his or her inheritance? Many things: parental overindulgence, feelings of being unloved, a long-standing family overemphasis on money, a lack of funds, or a lack of training in the pleasure there is in generosity and sharing with others. Simple selfishness and greed also exist. This is a difficult problem to rectify unless your child is motivated to discover the basis of his or her attitudes toward material possessions. Try to understand any part you may have played in shaping these attitudes and see what changes you can make in them. But also protect yourself financially and emotionally from capitulating to your child's demands. *Your estate is your own to disperse as you see fit.* If your son or daughter puts the pressure on, it may help to keep the provisions of your will secret. If your child is capable of maintaining some rationality in this area, however, it may be helpful to say exactly what you intend to do so that he or she can learn to live with it. The important thing is to be decisive and remain unintimidated by veiled or open threats, pressures, and pleadings focused upon your property.

In general, your children's emotional reactions toward your personal life are likely to run deep. They require your special attention if you are to avoid unnecessary alienation and hostility. Family councils and heart-to-heart talks can help enormously. But if all else fails, look for professional advice and try to get your children to join you. If they refuse, seek help by yourself, but make it clear to your children (and to yourself) that you are working toward their eventual acceptance of your new life.

PRENUPTIAL LEGAL PLANNING

For those of you who have decided on a marriage, prenuptial legal planning is advisable and often essential. Demand is growing for similar planning *after* marriage, known as "postnuptial" agreement. We will focus on only one important form of such planning, the prenuptial agreement or contract, also called a premarital or antenuptial agreement. (Do not confuse it with modern marriage contracts, which stipulate marital duties and are not legally binding.) Prenuptial agreements deal only with money and other property. You may also want to consider alternative forms (trusts, for example), but these are beyond the scope of this book. Whatever kind of prenuptial planning you elect will require consultation with a lawyer.

Many parents want to leave at least part of their estate directly to their children and become concerned about the effects of remarriage on this intention. If you are planning to remarry and want to make special financial arrangements for the benefit of your children or any other persons, you and your spouse-to-be can work out a prenuptial agreement. In most states these agreements are a time-honored method for allaying the fears of children and planning one's estate wisely and in their best interests. Such agreements also protect you by keeping your resources intact and unavailable to anyone but those whom you have designated. Wealthy people of all ages have traditionally used prenuptial agreements to protect their estates. Now, with people living longer, with more late-life marriages, and with more extensive estates to dispose of, prenuptial agreements are increasingly common. The agreement customarily describes what will *not* be available to the prospective spouse.

To be legally enforceable, such an agreement must be in writing, by reason of the Statute of Frauds in force in all states. The Uniform Premarital Agreement Act, approved by the American Bar Association in February 1984, can be used as a model for a premarital agreement. Since it is a basic agreement acceptable in all states, it is likely to stand up in court. For copies of the agreement, ask your lawyer or contact your local chapter of the American Bar Association.

How does a prenuptial agreement work? Let's take as an example a couple who plans to marry, each of whom has been widowed and has children. The prenuptial agreement enables them to plan their respective estates in the way that best suits them. The advantage to the children lies in the fact that their parent's new spouse will receive an amount less than ordinary under the Statute of Descent and Distributions and the children will receive more. An added advantage is that under such an agreement the children will receive somewhat more than if the parent had died intestate (without a will).

A prenuptial agreement *is* different from a will. It is a waiver to the right of the spouse to a certain minimum claim to your property at death. A will can be changed at any time without the spouse's knowledge or consent; a prenuptial agreement can be amended *only* with the consent of both parties. It is binding as soon as the marriage takes place; a will goes into effect only at the time of death. A will can, of course, be changed to give a spouse more and the children less than what the prenuptial agreement stated. But unless the will stipulates this, the spouse cannot lay claim to any more than what the prenuptial agreement provides for.

Prenuptial agreements are useful even though estates may be small. Take, as an example, a widower of moderate assets with children by his first wife, who had assisted him in earning the money he has accumulated and whose children contributed actively as well. Now that he wants to remarry, there is some resentment on the part of the children that the new bride will be automatically entitled to one-third (or whatever proportion is operative in a particular state) of their father's entire estate in the event of his death. If he chooses to do so, the father can decide on a prenuptial agreement that provides something less than one-third of the estate for the new wife, with the rest going to children or grandchildren. The financial gain to the children may be small, but emotionally it may mean a great deal.

There are situations where prenuptial agreements have been challenged, and the courts have in some cases upheld those challenges if fraud was involved or certain formalities had not been observed. The law says that the contracting parties must be in a confidential (or fiduciary) relationship to each other, meaning that there *must* be a good-faith disclosure of assets. For example, suppose a man who has several hundred thousand dollars tells his bride-to-be he has only twenty thousand dollars; she agrees on the basis of his statement to take the sum of five thousand dollars in the event of his death. His failure to reveal the truth makes the agreement subject to challenge on the basis of fraud.

Another problem arises from separation or divorce. Prenuptial agreements provide for the eventuality of death, and these agreements are expressly recognized in about one-fourth of the states by statute and in most of the other states by judicial decision. When the agreement deals not only with the division of property in the event of death, but with the possibility of divorce as well, you may encounter problems. For example, many states hold that agreements entered into before marriage to provide for divorce payments (in the event of separation) are invalid. However, a Washington, DC, District Court of Appeals decision (*Burtoff v. Burtoff*) upheld this broadening of a prenuptial agreement as it related to alimony and property settlements. Nonetheless, many agreements have been thrown out or modified by the courts after one of the parties has accused the other of coercion. To minimize such challenges, make certain that you draw up an agreement well in advance of the wedding, in order to avoid charges of duress. And *never* force such an agreement upon your partner. It must be a mutual understanding that both wish to participate.

So how much should you tell your children about your prenuptial agreement, or the making or changing of your will? Some parents inform each child fully or have their lawyer do so. Others give a general picture but not the specifics. Still others keep everything totally secret. What you do depends on your own judgment. Children may be relieved to have at least a general idea of your intentions. But if privacy about your own financial affairs is important to you, you have every right to keep the arrangements to yourself.

CHAPTER 12

❧ ❧

WHERE TO GO
FOR HELP

We have discussed throughout this book what older people can do for themselves to understand and remedy sexual, personal, and social problems. But when such problems persist, it is a good idea to seek outside professional help.

A thorough evaluation is crucial to determining exactly where the problem lies. And the first step in any evaluation of sexual problems in your age group should *always* be a medical examination. Physical problems can cause serious sexual difficulties by themselves, or they can team up with emotional or social problems to create quite a baffling group of sexual symptoms. Unraveling the medical aspects of sexual problems may be simple, or it may be terribly complicated; in either case, it should not be neglected.

FINDING MEDICAL HELP

How do you find a doctor who is knowledgeable about sex? More specifically, how do you find one who is interested in older people and who understands the special problems of sex in later life? Frankly, it may be very difficult. Many doctors—especially those graduating from medical school before 1961—have not had sex education as part of their medical school training. While this has slowly changed, you will still find that many doctors are surprisingly unenlightened and embarrassed to talk about sexual activity throughout the course of one's life. Many draw primarily upon their own personal sexual philosophy and experience. (This is especially true about sex in the later years.) They may also personally share the culture's negative attitude toward old age. It is not uncommon for women past fifty who see only an internist or a family practitioner (rather than a gynecologist) to find that their doctor begins to "forget" to do a thorough gynecological exam during a routine physical examination.

Adding to the difficulty of a search for a sympathetic

and knowledgeable doctor is the fact that most doctors have not had systematic training in the general medical problems of older people. This also is slowly changing and some medical school programs have begun to include geriatrics—the prevention, cure, and treatment of the problems of older people—in their curricula, but lack of knowledge and interest remains widespread among practicing physicians. Two national organizations, the American Geriatrics Society (The Empire State Building, 350 Fifth Avenue, Suite 801, New York, NY 10118, Phone: 212-308-1414) and the Gerontological Society of America's Clinical Medicine Section (1030 15th Street, N.W., Suite 250, Washington, DC 20005, Phone: 202-842-1275) may be able to help you locate doctors in your area who are knowledgeable in geriatrics. You can also contact the Office of Information of the National Institute on Aging (National Institutes of Health, Bethesda, MD 20892, Phone: 301-496-1752) or the National Institute of Mental Health (National Institutes of Health, Bethesda, MD 20892, Phone: 301-443-4513) for a list of doctors or clinics specializing in geriatrics and gerontology arranged by geographical area. After taking fellowship training and an exam, doctors can now obtain a Certificate of Competence in geriatrics, within the specialties of internal medicine, family practice, and psychiatry. Ask your doctor if he or she is so certified.

It is wise to remember that there are an extremely small percentage of doctors active in this field. It is also true that membership in geriatric and gerontological organizations does not guarantee competence in the field of aging, and individual doctors who are not specialists in the field may be equally sensitive and knowledgeable in working with older people. An able and understanding general practitioner or internist who takes care of patients of all ages can serve you very well indeed. If you are lucky, your own doctor may be such a person. Some people, of course, feel more comfortable talking about sexual problems with a new doctor who is a total stranger, and if this is the case with you, by all means do so. The main point is to go to a doctor with whom you feel as relaxed as possible and whom you trust to be both medically competent and generally receptive toward older people.

What else can you do? You owe it to yourself to learn how to give proper information and ask the right questions, and thus encourage your doctor to take your sexual problems seriously. It may be embarrassing to talk about what is on your mind, but don't let that stop you. Your experiences and problems are shared by many older people. Tell the doctor *exactly* what you are worried about. Include any detail that you think might be helpful in evaluating the symptoms. Older women may feel reluctant to describe sexual problems in general, or problems in the vaginal area in particular, especially to a male doctor. Older men may not want to admit problems with potency. But this is false modesty and false pride. Candid talk will go a long way toward making it easier to diagnose and treat your problem.

There are a number of things you should look for as you work with doctors:

- Beware of any doctor who quickly dismisses your sexual concerns with such comments as "What do you expect at your age?" "Go home and take a cold shower," "Stop worrying," or "Nothing can be done." Persist in your desire for help; if the doctor continues to be unresponsive, find a new doctor.
- Expect the doctor to take a good medical history, which includes a review of the body's systems and functions as well as a history of present and past illnesses. Specifically, the doctor should ask you about any changes you have observed in your genital organs, including in men any bowing of the penis and in women stress incontinence.
- Be aware that not only do diseases affect sexuality but also the proper control of disease may, in many instances, restore good sexual functioning.
- Expect the doctor to take a thorough sexual and marital history as well as a medical history. Questions are likely to cover the ways you and your partner feel about sex, its frequency

and pleasure, and any disagreements you may have. The doctor will also explore the impact of attitudes toward sex that you may have developed in childhood. You will find it valuable to share with your doctor the history of sexual experiences you may have had with people at other times. Male patients should be asked if they have problems with urination and with achieving and holding erections. They should be questioned as to whether they ever have erections as they wake up in the morning. Females should be questioned carefully as to whether they are having any pain during intercourse or any unusual soreness or bleeding, and whether they are lubricating adequately.

• The doctor should ask what drugs you are taking, both prescription and over-the-counter, and be able to explain the sexual side effects of each drug. It is sometimes possible to switch to equally effective drugs with fewer sexual side effects.

• If you have already had surgery on any sex organs, the doctor should be able to tell you if this is in any way affecting your sexuality. If surgery is planned, learn in advance about any possible sexual consequences. Do not be embarrassed to ask specific questions about anything that is troubling you.

- Discuss with your doctor a program of preventive health care. This should include attention to smoking, drinking, nutrition, exercise, rest, stress, and emotional problems.
- Using these questions and the doctor's reactions to you as a guide, and relying as well on your own common sense, if you feel your doctor's examination has been insufficient, talk to him or her openly about your misgivings. As a patient, you are entitled to satisfaction.
- Review insurance payment procedures with your doctor. Many types of diagnostic and treatment procedures are now reimbursable under insurance programs, including Medicare.
- Finally, your doctor should ask if you have any questions.

After the medical examination it should be fairly clear whether physical problems are the sole or, more likely, the partial cause of symptoms of sexual dysfunction and whether medical treatment is indicated. The point of the medical examination is to find out whether bodily changes are involved significantly or not at all; if they are not, or they have only a minor significance, the search for the causes of sexual problems must move to emotional or psychological areas.

FINDING PSYCHOLOGICAL HELP

Most sexual problems have emotional components, even when the original cause is physical, and some are entirely emotional in origin. Much of what we have said about the competence and inclinations of medical doctors with regard to older people also holds true for psychotherapists and counselors. They tend to be unaware of, and at times uninterested in, the emotional problems of later life. They have usually had some training in sex education but rarely in the specialized area of sex after sixty. To find a therapist who can be of help to you will probably require major determination.

The following is a classic humorous story that exposes some of the false assumptions about the elderly and their sexuality: A couple well into their eighties visited a sex therapist asking for a consultation. The therapist suggested that they might be at the wrong place and explained that his job was to help people with sexual problems. "But that's why we're here," the husband emphasized. The therapist proceeded to ask skeptically, "When was the first time you noticed this sexual problem?" "Why, last night," the wife replied matter-of-factly, "and then again this morning."

That said, there are several types of therapy from which to choose. *Individual psychotherapy* means talking

317

with a therapist one-to-one on a regular basis. *Marital counseling* involves both you and your partner. A broader term is *couples therapy*, which encompasses unmarried couples as well. *Family counseling* means the inclusion of other members of your family. *Psychoanalysis* is an intensive form of individual psychotherapy, requiring several sessions a week. *Group psychotherapy* usually consists of a group of five to ten patients whose problems are discussed by the group under the guidance of one or two therapists. *Cognitive therapy* aims at changing maladaptive patterns of thinking, feeling, and behavior. *Sex therapy* is a relatively new specialty, which concentrates on the actual sexual problem itself, teaching couples how to make love more effectively.

The background and training of therapists vary greatly. Psychotherapists can be *psychiatrists* (M.D.'s who specialize in psychiatry), *psychologists* (with master's or doctoral degrees in psychology), or *social workers* (with master's or doctoral degrees in social work). (The term *social worker* can be confusing, since people may define themselves as social workers because of the kind of work they do rather than because of their training. Ask if the social worker has, at minimum, a master's degree in social work.) *Psychoanalysts* have had advanced training in the psychoanalytic method. All these fields require a program of formal education and a supervised training period in psychotherapy or casework. All states require doctors to be licensed, and this is beginning to be true for practicing psychologists and social workers as well. Social workers who are certified (you will see the letters A.C.S.W.—for Academy of Certified Social Workers—after their names) by the National Association of Social Workers have had a period of professional training and examination beyond the master's degree. A number of states also have a special certification for advanced clinical social workers.

In addition to psychotherapists, there are numerous other kinds of counselors. *Marriage counselors* work with marriage and sex problems. This is a still unregulated field and practitioners range from competent and well-trained professionals to quacks and charlatans. Be careful to investigate the credentials (professional training and experience) of anyone you are considering as a counselor. *Pastoral counseling* has grown out of the counseling role of the clergy, with individual clerics counseling, supervising, and training others to counsel. The quality of this counseling depends on the training and skills of each individual; there are no standard requirements for such training in theological schools.

Well-trained *sex therapists* are usually much more able than other health professionals to evaluate and help resolve specific sexual problems. A general rule is that if you are seeing your family doctor, cleric, etc., regarding sexual problems, a resolution to your problems should begin to occur in six to eight sessions. If it doesn't you should seek referral to a specialist in sex therapy. *All about Sex Therapy*, by Peter R. Kilmann, M.D., and Katherine H. Mills, M.D. (Plenum Press, 1983), will help answer your questions about how sex therapy works.

Sex therapists have proliferated in recent years. Following Masters and Johnson's important clinical work in the treatment of sexual dysfunction, thousands of practitioners now offer such therapy. But many are untrained or poorly trained, and some are outright frauds. Because this is a somewhat recent field without an organized and uniform structure of qualifications, requirements, examinations, clinical experience, or peer review (licensing laws vary from state to state)—and because sexual problems are so susceptible to exploitation by skillful, smooth-talking incompetents—the choice of a sex counselor requires very careful consideration. Qualified sex therapists have basic backgrounds in psychotherapy and are licensed or certified by the state as a psychologist, psychiatrist, social worker, marriage and family therapist, professional counselor, or psychiatric nurse. They should have extensive training and experience in understanding human sexuality and treatment of sexual disorders.

How do you find competent psychotherapists, counselors, and sex therapists? Some sources to check are university medical schools and clinical teaching hospitals (many have sex therapy clinics); local medical or psychiatric societies; university schools of social work; community mental health centers; senior centers; local chapters of the National Association of Social Workers, Inc. (contact 750 First Street, N.E., Suite 700, Washington, DC 20002, Phone: 800-638-8799 for a listing of local chapters); the American Psychological Association (contact 750 First Street N.E., Washington, DC 20002, Phone: 800-374-2721 for a list of psychological associations in your state); the National Mental Health Association (contact 1021 Prince Street, Alexandria, VA 22314, Phone: 703-684-7722 for a list of local chapters); Family Service America (to find its member Family Service agencies, contact 11700 West Lake Park Drive, Milwaukee, WI 53224, Phone: 800-221-2681); and your family doctor or cleric.

When talking to these suggested sources, be specific and ask for a therapist who will be interested in working with an older person in sex counseling. Ask for at least two names so you will be able to make a choice. Friends and acquaintances may be able to refer you to professionals who have been helpful to them, as long as you recognize that individual preferences vary considerably.

The National Institute of Mental Health's Public Information Office (6001 Executive Boulevard, Room 8184, Bethesda, MD 20892, Phone: 301-443-4513) and the Gerontological Society's Social Research, Planning, and Practice Section (1030 15th Street, N.W., Suite 250, Washington, DC 20005, Phone: 202-842-1275) can be contacted for information. The American Association for Marriage and Family Therapy (1133 15th Street, N.W., Suite 300, Washington, DC 20005, Phone: 202-452-0109) is pressing for regulation of persons who call themselves marriage counselors and should be able to refer you to someone in your locale (including Canada). The American Association of Sex Educators, Counselors, and Therapists (AASECT) (P.O. Box 5488, Richmond, VA 23220) certifies sex counselor/therapists and has a national roster from which names can be obtained. You may want to write the Masters and Johnson Institute (16216 Baxter Road, Suite 399, St. Louis, MO 63017, Phone: 636-532-9772) for referral to competent sex counselors near you who have been trained by them. The Sexuality Information and Education Council of the United States (SIECUS) (130 West 42nd, Suite 350, New York, NY 10036-7802, Phone: 212-819-9770 and 1638 R Street N.W., Suite 220, Washington, DC 20009, Phone: 202-265-2405) is an additional source of information and referral.

The cost of therapy varies from free clinics and free counseling, to sliding fees based on income, up to $250 or more for a fifty-minute session (in 2000). Group therapy is less costly than individual therapy. Some health insurance plans partially cover costs of psychotherapy. Many do not. Medicare now pays 50 percent of the allowable charge for psychotherapy, whether performed by physicians, psychologists, or social workers. Medicare will also cover some of the costs of a physical evaluation for sexual dysfunction, but not outpatient medications such as Viagra. Some private insurance companies, including some Medicare supplementary plans, cover prescription drugs like Viagra, antidepressants, and the like. Few plans cover sex therapy per se. However, the Diagnostic and Statistical Manual of Mental Disorders (DSM-IV-R) categorizes sexual dysfunctions under the following: Sexual Desire Disorders; Sexual Arousal Disorders; Orgasm Disorders; and Sexual Pain Disorders. Some insurance companies will reimburse if a specific DSM-IV-R diagnosis is used. So ask your therapist if such a diagnosis may be relevant for you and you may be reimbursed for at least part of your costs.

The amount of time required for evaluating and, if possible, resolving a particular sexual problem varies. Sometimes a single session can be enough. More often a series of weekly sessions is recommended, lasting from several months to more than a year or, in the case of psychoanalysis, a number of years.

WHAT HAPPENS IN PSYCHOTHERAPY?

You can't, literally, change the past, obviously, but you can gain perspective about it, change the way you feel about it, and break old habits and acquire new ways of coping effectively. Through talking about and exploring your past patterns, you come to understand the sources of sexual problems, lose certain inhibitions, and learn new avenues of sexual expression. Therapeutic counseling does not simply dwell on the past, however. You will also be discussing the here and now, your present relationships. Your therapist will ask questions, make comments (some may startle you), and propose suggestions. Working out conflicts and going in new directions, therefore, come about through joint work by you *and* your therapist on the past and the present. Together you work on your private life.

The process itself may remind you of both parenting and teaching. You retain your basic personality, but hopefully you rid yourself of unwelcome symptoms, gain insight and enhanced well-being, and increase your effectiveness in everyday living. Altogether you are likely to feel better about yourself.

How should you act when you go to the therapist? Once again, be frank. Tell him or her whatever is troubling you. There are certain basic things you can require or expect:

- Your therapist needs to be well informed both about the problems of older people and about sexual problems. Don't be afraid to question therapists about their background, training, and general interest in these areas. Evaluate their answers (or failures to answer) in terms of what you now know—from this book and from your own experiences—to be important to you.

- The therapist should ask for your sexual, marital, and personal history, and probably will want a medical report from your doctor.
- You should feel a sense of rapport and comfort with the therapist by the time you have had several sessions. If not, discuss your feelings frankly. If matters do not improve, you may need to consider a different therapist, since rapport and trust are crucial to effectively working out sexual and emotional problems. However, do not consider the need to change therapists to be the result of a flaw in yourself. Each individual's requirements in a relationship as close as that of therapist and patient will be different, and intangible but crucial factors like empathy, perception, manner, and attitude are involved in making the right choice. A personality and approach that are right for one person may be all wrong for another. As long as you are candid in your encounters with the therapist, trust in your own perceptions about whether he or she is a good choice for you.

As for your part in the therapy, you must learn to:

- Set aside shyness and embarrassment.
- Open your mind and feelings to new ideas and insights.

- Be willing to actively try new directions in your relationships with others.
- Realize that while many things can improve, some things cannot. Once you have decided—with the aid of your therapist—which is which, you can begin to work on those areas where improvement can realistically occur.

WHAT HAPPENS IN SEX THERAPY?

Sex therapy is a unique, usually short-term form of therapy that has evolved over the past thirty years under the leadership of Dr. William Masters and Virginia Johnson of St. Louis. This method is quite effective in rapidly treating problems like premature ejaculation, vaginal spasm, failure to achieve orgasm, and some forms of impotence. It is much more difficult, but not always impossible, to treat low or absent sexual desire or lack of pleasure in sex. (Low sexual desire usually requires longer-term and more intensive psychotherapy.) "Desire discrepancy," which occurs when one partner wishes to have sex more (or less) frequently than the other, is another common problem that can often be resolved in this kind of therapy.

The original Masters and Johnson sex therapy techniques required a male and female therapist for each couple, a two-week stay in a hotel near the treatment center (so the couple was isolated and could concentrate on therapy), and daily therapy sessions. Patients were provided with two years of follow-up assistance from therapists available twenty-four hours a day (usually by telephone), for no extra charge. Most sex therapists now have modified this so that couples can remain in their own communities and homes and have therapy once or twice a week for about fourteen sessions. Educational counseling about sex, improving communication between a couple, and carrying out "pleasuring exercises" are all part of treatment.

Therapists may use movies and slides in their teaching, as well as group therapy. Couples with marital problems that go beyond their sexual difficulties are encouraged to obtain marital counseling and/or individual psychotherapy. Also, you should know that individuals who are not part of a couple are also accepted for sex therapy.

In summary, we'd like to make very clear that even sexual problems that have existed for many years have the possibility of resolution. This is true whether your current relationship is new or long-term. If your sexual functioning is troubling to you, you owe it to yourself to see what can be done to resolve your concerns. In many cases you will be happy with the results.

CHAPTER 13

❧❧❧

LOVE AND LIFE AS A WORK OF ART

Can sex really remain interesting and exciting after forty, fifty, or sixty years of adulthood? Yes. Older people themselves have testified that it can. Affection, warmth, and sensuality do not have to deteriorate with age; they may, in fact, increase.

Sex in later life is sex for its own sake: pleasure, release, communication, shared intimacy. Except for older men involved with younger women, it is no longer associated with childbearing and the creation of families. This freedom can be both exhilarating and insightful, especially for those who have literally never had the time until now to think about and get to know themselves and each other.

Love and sex can mean many different things to older people:

- *The opportunity for expression of passion, affection, admiration, loyalty, and other positive emotions.* This can occur in long-term relationships that have steadily grown and developed over the years, in relationships that actually improve in later years, and in new relationships such as second or third marriages.
- *An affirmation of one's body and its functioning.* An active sex life demonstrates to older people that their bodies are still capable of working well and providing pleasure. For many people, satisfactory sexual functioning is an extremely important part of their lives and helps to maintain high morale and enthusiasm.
- *A strong sense of self.* Sexuality is one of the ways people get a sense of their identity—who they are and what their impact is on others. Positive reactions from others preserve and enhance our self-esteem. Feeling "feminine" or "masculine," whatever meaning these terms have for each individual, is connected with feeling valued as a person. Negative reactions depress and discourage older people and may tempt them to write off their sexuality forever.

- *A means of self-assertion.* The patterns of self-assertion available when people are young change as they grow older. Their children are grown-up and gone; their jobs are usually behind them; personal and social relationships now become far more important as outlets for expressing personality. Sex can be a valuable means of positive self-assertion. One man told us, "I feel like a million dollars when I make love even though we are scrimping along on Social Security. My wife has always made me feel like a great success in bed and I believe I do the same for her. We've been able to stand a lot of stress in life because of our closeness this way."

- *Protection from anxiety.* The intimacy and the closeness of sexual union bring security and significance to people's lives, particularly when the outside world threatens them with hazards and losses. An older couple we know described the warmth of their sexual life as "a port in the storm," a place to escape from worry and trouble. A very much older woman, concerned with her eventual death, called sex "the ultimate closeness against the night." Sex serves as an important means of feeling in charge when other elements of one's life feel out of control.

- *Defiance of the stereotypes of aging.* Familiar though they are with the derogatory attitudes

of society toward late-life sex, older people
who are sexually active defy the neutered status expected of them. We have heard them say,
"We're not finished yet," "I'm not ready to
kick the bucket," "You can't keep a good man
[woman] down," or "There may be snow on
the roof but there's still fire in the furnace."
And it's true.

- *The pleasure of being touched or caressed.* Older
  widows, widowers, and divorced people describe how much they miss the simple pleasure and warmth of physical closeness, of
  being touched, held, and caressed by someone
  they care for. Holding and hugging friends,
  children, and pets offer some compensation
  but do not replace the special intimacy and
  feeling of being cared about that can exist in a
  good relationship or sexual union.

- *A sense of romance.* The courting aspects of
  sexuality may be highly significant—flowers,
  soft lights, music, a sense of romantic pursuit,
  elegance, sentiment, and courtliness—and give
  pleasure in themselves. Romance may continue even when sexual intercourse, for various reasons, ceases. John and Rachel, a couple
  in their eighties, described their evenings together to us. They typically bathe and dress for
  dinner, she in a long dress, he in a suit and tie.
  They dine with candlelight and music, listen to

music during the evening, hold hands, and enjoy each other's companionship. At bedtime they fall asleep in each other's arms. Often they awaken in the middle of the night and have long, intimate conversations, sleeping late the next morning. John said of his wife, "I fall in love with her every day. My feelings grow stronger when I realize we have only a certain amount of time left."

• *An affirmation of life.* Sex expresses joy and continued affirmation of life. The quality of one's most intimate relationships is an important measure of whether life has been worthwhile. Many otherwise successful people may count their lives a failure if they have been unable to achieve significant closeness to other people, and have never felt fully desired or accepted. Conversely, people with modest accomplishments may feel highly satisfied about themselves if they have been affirmed through intimate relationships. Sexual intimacy is only one way of achieving intimacy, of course, but it is an especially profound affirmation of the worthwhileness of life.

• *A continuing search for sensual growth and experience.* Some older people continue to search throughout their lives for ways to create new excitement and experiences. Some who are dissatisfied with their present lives look for ways to improve them. Others seek marriage counseling, pursue divorce, remarriage, or new relationships in the hope of finding what they are searching for. But many can find this growth and excitement within their present relationship if they learn some of the skills that make it possible. Love and sex are twin arts: both require effort and knowledge. Only in fairy tales do people live happily ever after without working at it. It takes a continuous and active effort to both master the processes that eradicate emotional distances between two people and to continue to grow and learn.

When people are young and first getting used to sexuality, their sex tends to be urgent and explosive. It is involved largely with physical pleasure and in many cases the conception of children. This is the *first language of sex*. It is biological and instinctive, wonderfully exciting and energizing. The process of discovering one's ability to be sexually desirable and sexually effective often becomes a way of asserting independence, strength, prowess, and power. The first language of sex has been much discussed and written about because it is easy to study and measure; one can tabulate physical response, frequency of contacts, forms of outlet, sexual positions, and physical skills in lovemaking. But sex is not just a matter of athletics and "production." Some people recognize this early on and simultaneously develop a *second language of sex*, which is emotional and communicative as well as physical. Others continue largely in the first language—sometimes all their lives, sometimes only until they begin to see its limitations and desire something more.

The second language is largely learned rather than instinctive and is often vastly underdeveloped, since it depends upon the ability to recognize and share feelings in words, actions, and unspoken perceptions, and to achieve mutual tenderness and thoughtfulness with another person. In its richest form, the second language becomes highly creative and imaginative, with bountiful possibilities for new emotional experiences. Yet, it is a slow-developing aptitude, acquired deliberately and painstakingly through years of experience in giving and receiving. Eleanor Roosevelt once observed, "Beautiful young people are accidents of nature, beautiful old people are works of art."

In the natural flow of events in the life cycle, you will eventually find yourself reevaluating many areas of your life, including your sexuality. Middle age is the period when people typically begin to take stock of their lives and reassess their work, their personal relationships, and their social and spiritual commitments. Retirement is another time when such reevaluations take place. Both periods can be chaotic, generating emotional upsets, divorce, a higher risk of alcoholism, and other evidences of stress.

But these can be constructive as well as dangerous ages, and the second language of sex has a good deal to offer you if you want to move in new directions in your personal life. Shared tenderness, warmth, humor, merriment, anger, passion, sorrow, camaraderie, fear— feelings of every conceivable sort can flow back and forth in a sexual relationship that has matured to this level of development.

Part of the secret of learning the second language lies in learning how to give. Receiving is much easier. It makes few demands. But the habit of only taking deadens the impulse to reciprocate. As Erich Fromm wrote in *The Art of Loving* (1956), "Most people see the problem of love primarily as that of being loved, rather than that of loving, of one's capacity to love." Giving is not an endless gift of yourself to others in which you expect nothing in return. Nor is it a marketplace transaction, trading with the expectation of an equal exchange. Healthy giving involves not only the hopeful and human anticipation that something equally good will be returned but also the pleasures inherent in giving, regardless of the return. The balance to be struck must be chosen by each person and worked out in partnership.

The second language implies sensitivity. It means clearing up long-held grudges and old irritations toward your partner and people in general so that your energy is

not wasted in negativity. It suggests the possibility of re-
newing love every day. It requires knowing what pleases
your partner and what pleases you. It involves playful-
ness as well as passion, and talking, laughing, teasing,
sharing secrets, reminiscing, telling jokes, making plans,
confessing fears and uncertainties, crying—all in the privacy of shared companionship. In fact, it need not involve the sex act at all.

If boredom creeps into the relationship, both you
and your partner need to acknowledge it; it is time to
look for, or listen to, the deeper feelings that each of you
has hidden away against the time when the richness of
such feelings will be welcome and restorative. You have
to *resist* the pulls of habit. Routines and responsibilities
may have dulled the impulse to really talk; fight against
succumbing to the temptation to withdraw into your
own self-absorbed world. Self-centeredness, wanting
sexual and emotional contact only when you are in the
mood, without concern for your partner's needs, is guaranteed to produce conflict. Competitiveness based on
some fancied level of sexual performance is also deadly.

The second language of sex can be developed by
actively trying to learn it. Older people may have struggled throughout their lives to overcome obstacles, earn a
living, raise a family, and carry out other responsibilities.
In doing so they have literally sacrificed their private
lives and individual growth to this process. But fortunately love and sex are *always* there, waiting to be redis-
covered, enhanced, or even appreciated for the very first

time, whether you are young or very old. Self-starters have the advantage over those who wait passively for love to strike like lightning.

Older people have, in fact, a special ability to bring love and sex to new levels of development because they are more experienced. Many people do learn from experience. They develop perceptions that are connected with the unique sense of having lived a long time and having struggled to come to terms with life as a cycle from birth to death. A number of these qualities are beautifully suited to the flourishing of the second language. An appreciation of the preciousness of life and the valuing of immediateness can occur as people become older. What counts now is the present moment, where once it was the casually expected future. If developing an awareness of the brevity of life leads you to come to terms with your own mortality in a mature and healthy way, by no longer denying it, you will find you no longer live heedlessly, as though you had all the time in the world. The challenge of living as richly as possible in the time you have left can be exhilarating, not depressing.

Elementality—the enjoyment of the elemental things of life—may develop in late life precisely because older people are more keenly aware that life is short. Such people may find themselves becoming more adept in separating out the important from the trivial. They might uncover a heightened responsiveness to nature, human warmth, children, music, and beauty in any form. Healthy late life is frequently a time for greater enjoyment of all the senses—colors, sights, sounds, smells, touch—and less involvement with the transient drives for achievement, possessions, and power.

Older people have time for love. Although they have fewer years left to live than the young and middle-aged, if they are in reasonably good health they can often spend more time on social and sexual relationships than any other age group. It is true that many have limited financial resources, but fortunately social and personal relationships are among the pleasures in life that can be free of charge.

Willingness to change counts as well. It is possible to become quite different in later life from what you were in youth. Obviously, the change can go in positive or negative directions. But the point to remember is that *change is possible.* You do not need to become locked into any particular mode of behavior at any time of life. Experimentation and learning are possible all throughout your life, and this holds true for both sex and love. Naturally, the more actively you grow, the greater the reservoir of experience and the larger the repertoire you can draw upon in getting along with and loving other people.

The early and middle years set the stage, but perhaps only in the later years can life, with its various choices and possibilities, have the chance to shape itself into something approximating a human work of art. And perhaps only in later life, when your personality reaches its final stages of development, can lovemaking and sex achieve the fullest possible growth. Sex does not merely *exist* in the later years; it can become greater than it ever was.

The special psychology of sex in the second half of life will eventually be better understood than it is now. Then we will comprehend for the first time the full life cycle of love and sexuality—with youth a time for exciting exploration and self-discovery; middle age, for gaining skill, confidence, and discrimination; and old age, for bringing the experience of a lifetime and the unique perspectives of the final years of life to the art of loving one another. We have a great deal yet to learn from those who personally have mastered this complex and wonderful art over years of time.

GLOSSARY

androgen Any of the *steroid** hormones produced by the adrenal glands, the *testes*, and also the ovaries, that develop and maintain masculine characteristics; *testosterone* is the best known.

anus The opening from the lower bowel (colon) through which solid waste is passed.

atrophy A wasting away or diminution in size of a cell, tissue, organ, part, or body.

Bartholin's glands Two small, roundish bodies, one on either side of the vaginal opening. Although they produce mucus in sexual excitement, they are not

---

*Italicized words are defined elsewhere in the Glossary.

the primary source of vaginal lubrication during intercourse.

benign prostatic hypertrophy (BPH)   Noncancerous enlargement of the *prostate* gland that occurs in the middle and later years.

bladder   The distendable elastic sac that serves as a receptacle and place of storage for the urine.

cervix   The part of the *uterus*, sometimes called the neck, which protrudes into the *vagina*.

circumcision   Surgical removal of the foreskin, a loose fold of skin that surrounds the head of the penis.

climacteric   See **menopause**.

climax   See **orgasm**.

clitoris   A small, erectile organ at the upper end of the *vulva*, homologous with the *penis*, and a significant focus of sexual excitement and *orgasm* in the woman.

coitus   Copulation, coition, sexual intercourse.

Cowper's glands   A pair of small glands lying alongside and discharging into the male *urethra*. They contribute lubrication during sexual activity.

cystitis   Inflammation of the urinary bladder.

dyspareunia   The occurrence of pain in the sexual act, usually experienced in the female vaginal area.

ejaculation   The forceful emission of the seminal fluid at *orgasm*.

ejaculatory impotence   Inability to ejaculate.

erectile dysfunction   Problems with penile erection, which prevent copulation. See **impotence**.

erogenous zones   Sensitive areas of the body, such as the mouth, lips, buttocks, breasts, and genital areas, which are important in sexual arousal.

estrogen   One of the active female hormones produced by the *ovaries*, the adrenal glands, and also the testes, which has a profound effect on the generative organs and breasts.

Fallopian tube   The tube that leads from each *ovary* into the *uterus*; after *ovulation* the ovum travels through the tube on its way to the *uterus* and fertilization takes place in the tube.

flashes (or flushes), hot   A symptom associated with the hormonal changes during *menopause*, caused by a sudden rapid dilation of blood vessels.

foreplay   Sexual acts which precede intercourse, during which the partners stimulate each other by kissing, touching, and caressing.

frigidity   An imprecise term applied to various aspects of female sexual inadequacy: (1) popularly, abnormal lack of desire, or coldness; (2) inability to achieve an *orgasm* through intercourse; (3) inability to achieve *orgasm* by any means; (4) any other level of sexual response considered unsatisfactory by the woman or her partner.

genital area   The area which contains the external genital organs such as the *vulva* in the female and the *penis* and scrotum in the male.

genitalia   The reproductive organs, especially the external organs.

hormones Chemical substances produced in the ductless (endocrine) glands of the body and discharged directly into the bloodstream. They have specific effects upon the activity of a certain organ or organs. Sexual hormones regulate the entire reproductive cycle. (The body produces many nonsexual hormones as well.)

hormone replacement therapy (HRT) The medical use of supplementary hormones (other than, or in addition to, those produced by the endocrine glands) for treatment of diseases and deficiencies.

impotence See **erectile dysfunction**.

intimacy Close emotional, empathetic relationship.

labia Two rounded folds of tissue that form the outer boundaries of the external genitals in the female.

libido Sexual desire.

mastectomy Surgical removal of a breast.

masturbation Stimulation of the sex organs, usually to *orgasm*, through manual or mechanical means.

medical specialties regarding sex:

    endocrinology The functions and diseases of the ductless (endocrine) glands.

    gynecology The diseases, reproductive functions, organs, and endocrinology of females.

    urology The functions, organs, and diseases of the urinary system in males and females and of the reproductive system in males.

menopause The time of life for the human female, usually between the ages of forty-five and fifty-five, which is marked by the cessation of *menstruation* and *ovulation*. It may be gradual or sudden, and it can last from three months to three years, or even longer. It marks the end of the childbearing potential.

menstruation The periodic discharge of the body fluid (menses) from the *uterus* through the *vagina*, occurring normally once a month.

nocturnal emission *Ejaculation* of *semen* at night while asleep; often called a wet dream.

oral-genital sex Forms of stimulation of the *genitalia* by the mouth:

cunnilingus Stimulation of the *vulva* (especially the *clitoris* and *labia*) by the partner's mouth and tongue.

fellatio Stimulation of the *penis* by the partner's mouth and tongue.

orchiectomy (orchidectomy) Removal of one or both *testes*; castration.

orgasm The culmination of the sex act. There is a feeling of sudden, intense pleasure accompanied by an abrupt increase in pulse rate and blood pressure. Involuntary spasms of pelvic muscles cause relief of sexual tension with vaginal contractions in the female and *ejaculation* by the male. It lasts up to ten seconds.

ovaries The two major reproductive glands of the female, in which the ova (eggs) are formed and *estrogen*, or female hormones, are produced.

ovulation The process in which a mature egg is discharged by an *ovary* for possible fertilization.

Papanicolaou test or Papanicolaou smear (Pap test) A simple test to determine the presence of cancer of the *uterus* by analyzing cells taken from the *cervix* or *vagina*.

penis The male organ of sexual intercourse.

perineum (1) The internal portion of the body in the pelvis occupied by urogenital passages and the rectum; (2) the internal and external region between the *scrotum* and *anus* in the man, and the *vulva* and *anus* in the woman.

pituitary gland An endocrine gland consisting of three lobes, located at the base of the brain. The body's master gland, it controls the other endocrine glands and influences growth, metabolism, and maturation.

potency Sexual capacity for intercourse; the ability to achieve and sustain erection. Applied only to the male.

premature ejaculation Almost instant *ejaculation* (within three seconds) upon entry of the *penis* into the *vagina*.

prostate A walnut-sized body, partly muscular and partly glandular, which surrounds the base of the urethra in the male. It secretes a milky fluid which is discharged into the *urethra* at the time of emission of *semen*.

prostatectomy Surgical removal of part or all of the

prostate. There are three types, depending upon the anatomical approach: (1) transurethral (TUR); (2) suprapubic (or retropubic); and (3) perineal.

prostatism, prostatitis Inflammation or congestion in the prostate.

refractory period See **sexual response cycle**.

replacement therapy See **hormone replacement therapy**.

scrotum The sac containing the *testes.*

semen The whitish fluid containing sperm, which is discharged in *ejaculation.*

sensuality The wider aspect of *sexuality*; the involvement of all the physical senses that enhance and express one's sexuality.

sex (1) Urge for, and (2) act of sexual union.

sexual dysfunction A general term for different varieties and degrees of unsatisfying sexual response and performance.

sexual fantasies Vivid and excitatory imaginings about sex; healthy and common in both sexes.

sexual hormones See **hormones**.

sexual response cycle The physical changes that occur in the body during sexual excitement and *orgasm.* It includes four phases: (1) the excitement or erotic-arousal phase during *foreplay*; (2) the intromission or plateau phase; (3) the orgasmic or climax phase; and (4) the resolution or recovery phase. The time required for the completion of recovery—the time required before the first phase can be successfully initiated again—is called the *refractory period*. The *refractory period* is more critical to the male.

sexuality The emotional and physical responsiveness to sexual stimuli. Also, one's sexual identity, role, and perception; one's femininity; one's masculinity.

sperm Spermatozoa, the male reproductive cells, produced by the *testes* and discharged during intercourse into the *vagina*.

sterility The incapacity to reproduce sexually; infertility.

steroids A class of chemical substances that includes the *sex hormones*.

testes (testicles) The two male reproductive glands, located in the cavity of the *scrotum*, the source of spermatozoa and the androgens.

testosterone A male hormone (an *androgen*), a *steroid*, produced by the testes.

thyroid gland The gland partially surrounding the windpipe (trachea) in the neck whose function is to supply *hormones* that adjust the metabolism of the body.

urethra The passage or canal in the *penis* through which the male discharges both urine and *sperm*. In women the passage through which urine passes.

urethritis Inflammation of the *urethra*.

urogenital system The organs that serve the functions of urination, sexual activity, and procreation.

uterus (womb) The hollow muscular organ in the female in which the embryo and fetus develop to maturity.

vagina The tube or sheath leading from the *uterus* to the *vulva* at the exterior of the body. It receives the *penis* during intercourse.

vaginitis Inflammation of the *vagina*.

vas deferens The duct from each *testicle* that carries *sperm* to the *penis*.

venereal disease Any disease that is transmitted during sexual activity.

virility Masculine vigor, including *potency* (from which it must be distinguished), sexual prowess (skill), sexual frequency, and attractiveness.

vulva The external female genitalia, including the *labia*, *clitoris*, and the outer *vagina*.

womb See **uterus**.

BIBLIOGRAPHY

Barbach, Lonnie. *For Yourself: The Fulfillment of Female Sexuality*. Garden City, NY: New American Library, 1991.

Boston Women's Health Collective. *Our Bodies, Ourselves for the New Century: A Book by and for Women*. New York: Touchstone Books, 1998.

Brecher, Edward M., and the Editors of *Consumer Reports Books*. *Love, Sex and Aging*. Boston: Little, Brown and Co., 1984.

Butler, Robert N., and Myrna I. Lewis. "Sexuality and Aging." In *Principles of Geriatric Medicine and Gerontology*, 4th Ed. Hazzard, W. R., Blass, J. P., Ettinger, W. H., Halter, J. B., and Ostander, J. G., Editors. New York: McGraw-Hill, 1999.

Butler, Robert N., and Myrna I. Lewis. "Sexuality." In *The Merck Manual of Geriatrics*, 3rd Ed. 2000.

Butler, Robert N., and Myrna I. Lewis. "Sexuality in Old Age." In *Brocklehurst's Textbook of Geriatric Medicine and Gerontology*. Edinburgh: Churchill Livingstone, 2002.

Carson, C., Jordan, G. H., and Gelbard, M. K. "Peyronie's Disease: New Concepts in Etiology, Diagnosis, and Treatment." *Contemporary Urology* (1999): 11:44.

Carson, Culley, Roger Kirby, and Irwin Goldstein. *Textbook of Erectile Dysfunction*. Oxford: Isis Medical Media Ltd., 1999.

Comfort, Alex. *The Joy of Sex*. New York: Crown, 1972.

———. ed. *Sexual Consequences of Disability*. Philadelphia: Stickley, 1978.

———. "Menopause: A Guide to Smart Choices." *Consumer Reports*. (January 1999): 48–54.

———. "When Sex and Drugs Don't Mix." *Consumer Reports on Health*. Consumers Union of the United States (December 1998): 9.

Curry, Hayden (Editor), Denis Clifford, Frederick Hertz, and Robin Leonard. *A Legal Guide for Lesbian and Gay Couples*. Berkeley, CA: Nolo Press, 1999.

Derogatis, L. R., and Conklin-Powers, B. "Psychological Assessment Measures of Female Sexual Functioning in Clinical Trials." *International Journal of Impotence Research* 10:S111–S1116, 1998.

Feldman, H. A. et al. "Impotence and Its Medical and

Psychosocial Correlates: Results of the Massachusetts Male Aging Study." *Journal of Urology* 151 (1994): 54.

Fromm, Erich. *The Art of Loving.* New York: HarperCollins (Harper & Row), 1956.

Gay, Peter, *The Bourgeois Experience: Victoria to Freud.* Vol. 1, *Education of the Senses.* New York: Oxford University Press, 1984.

Goldstein, Irwin, Tom F. Lue, Harin Padma-Nathan, Raymond C. Rosen, William D. Steers, and Pierre A. Wicker. (Sildenafil Study Group). "Oral Sildenafil in the Treatment of Erectile Dysfunction." *The New England Journal of Medicine* (1998): 338:1397–1404.

Goldstein, Irwin, M.D. and Larry Rothstein. *The Potent Male: Facts, Fiction, Future.* Los Angeles: Price, Stern Sloan, 1990.

Gottman, John. *Why Marriages Succeed or Fail: And How You Can Make Yours Last.* New York: Fireside, 1995.

Greenwald, Morgan. "The SAGE Model for Serving Older Lesbians and Gay Men." In *Homosexuality and Social Work,* 53–61. New York: Haworth Press, 1984.

Greenwood, Sadja. *Menopause Naturally: Preparing for the Second Half of Life.* Volcano, CA: Volcano Press, 1988.

Hammond, C. B. "Menopause and Hormone Replacement Therapy: An Overview." *Obstetrics and Gynecology,* 87 (1996): 25.

Hammond, Doris B. *My Parents Never Had Sex: Myths and Facts of Sexual Aging.* Buffalo, NY: Prometheus Books, 1988.

Heiman, Julia, and Joseph LoPiccolo. *Becoming Orgasmic: A Sexual Growth Program for Women.* Englewood Cliffs, NJ: Prentice-Hall, 1988.

International Longevity Center. *Prescription for Longevity: Fads and Reality.* New York: International Longevity Center, 1997.

International Longevity Center. *Maintaining Healthy Lifestyles: A Lifetime of Choices.* New York: International Longevity Center, 2000.

International Longevity Center. *Achieving and Maintaining Cognitive Vitality with Aging.* New York: International Longevity Center, 2001.

Isensee, Rik. *Love between Men: Enhancing Intimacy and Keeping Your Relationship Alive.* Boston: Alyson Publications, 1996.

Janus, Samuel S., and Cynthia L. Janus. *The Janus Report on Sexual Behavior.* New York: John Wiley & Sons, 1994.

Kaplan, Helen Singer. *Disorders of Sexual Desire and Other New Concepts and Techniques in Sex Therapy.* New York: Bruner/Mazel, 1979.

Kehoe, Monika. *Lesbians over Sixty Speak for Themselves.* New York: Hamington Park Press, 1989.

Kelly, James J. "The Aging Male Homosexual: Myth and Reality." In M. Levine, ed., *Sociology of Male Homosexuality,* 253–262. New York: Basic Books, 1979.

Kievman, Beverly, and Susie Blackman. *For Better or Worse: A Couple's Guide to Dealing with Chronic Illness.* Chicago: Contemporary Books, 1990.

Kinsey, Alfred C., Wardell Pomeroy, and Clyde E. Martin. *Sexual Behavior in the Human Male.* Reprint Edition. Bloomington, IN: Indiana University Press, 1998.

Kinsey, Alfred C., Wardell Pomeroy, Clyde E. Martin, and Paul M. Gebhard. *Sexual Behavior in the Human Female.* Reprint Edition. Bloomington, IN: Indiana University Press, 1998.

Kroll, K., and E. Levy-Klein. *Enabling Romance: A Guide to Love, Sex and Relationships for the Disabled.* New York: Harmony Books, 1992.

Laumann, E. O., A. Paik, and R. C. Rosen. "Sexual Dysfunction in the United States: Prevalence and Predictors." *Journal of the American Medical Association* 281 (1999): 537–544.

Leiblum, Sandra, and Raymond Rosen, Eds. *Principles and Practice of Sex Therapy: Update for the 1990s.* New York: Guilford, 1989.

Levin, Rhoda. Heartmates: *A Survival Guide for the Cardiac Spouse.* Minneapolis, MN: Minerva Press, 1994.

Lewis, R. W., and R. Witherington. "External Vacuum Therapy for Erectile Dysfunction: Use and Results." *World Journal of Urology* 15 (1997): 78–82.

Linet, O. I., and F. G. Ogrinc. "Efficacy and Safety of Intracavernosal Alprostadil in Men with Erectile

Dysfunction." The Aprostadil Study Group. *New England Journal of Medicine* 334 (1996): 873–877.

Masters, William H., and Virginia E. Johnson. *Human Sexual Response*. Boston: Little, Brown and Co., 1966.

————. *Human Sexual Inadequacy*. Boston: Little, Brown and Co., 1970.

Masters, William, Virginia Johnson, and R. Kolodny. *Masters and Johnson on Sex and Human Loving*. Boston: Little, Brown and Co., 1986.

McCullough, A. R. "Management of Erectile Dysfunction Following Radical Prostatectomy." *Sexual Dysfunction in Medicine* 2(1): 2–8, 2001.

Money, John. *Gay, Straight, and In Between*. New York: Oxford University Press, 1988.

Muller, J. E., Mittleman, A., Maclure, M., Sherwood, J. B., and Tofler, G. H. "Triggering Myocardial Infarction by Sexual Activity. Low Absolute Risk and Prevention by Regular Physical Exertion." *Journal of The American Medical Association* 275 (18): 1405–9, 1996.

Nachtigall, Lila E., and Joan R. Heilman. *Estrogen: A Complete Guide to Menopause and Hormone Replacement Therapy*. New York: HarperResource, 2000.

Napier, Augustus. *The Fragile Bond: In Search of an Equal, Intimate, and Enduring Marriage*. New York: HarperCollins, 1988.

National Council on the Aging. Booklets titled 1) *Sex: A Natural Part of Your Life*, 2) *Sexual Challenges and*

Solutions, and 3) *Talking to Your Doctor About Sex.* Pfizer, Inc., 1999.

National Council on the Aging. *Healthy Sexuality and Vital Aging: A Study by the National Council on the Aging.* September 1998.

National Institute on Aging. *Exercise: A Guide from the National Institute on Aging* (49-minute video and 100-page book). Bethesda, MD: National Institute on Aging, Pub. # NIH 99-4258, November 2000.

National Institutes of Health. "Consensus Development Panel on Impotence." *Journal of the American Medical Association* 270 (1993).

Norwinski, Joseph. *A Lifelong Love Affair: Keep Sexual Desire Alive in Your Relationship.* New York: Dodd, Mead, 1988.

Papadoupoulos, Chris. *Sexual Aspects of Cardiovascular Disease.* New York: Praeger, 1990.

Reinisch, June. *The Kinsey Institute New Report on Sex: What You Must Know to Be Sexually Literate.* New York: St. Martin's Press, 1990.

Richardson, J. P., and D. Lazur. "Sexuality and the Nursing Home Patient." *American Family Physician.* 51 (1995): 121.

Rosen, R. C., Taylor, J. F., Leiblum, S. R., and Bachmann, G. A. "Prevalence of Sexual Dysfunction in Women: Results of a Survey Study of 329 Women in an Outpatient Gynecological Clinic." *Journal of Sex and Marital Therapy* 19 (1993): 171–188.

Rosen, R. "Effects of SSRIs on Sexual Function: A

Critical Review." *Journal of Clinical Psychopharma-cololgy* 19 (1999): 65–67.

Rothman, Ellen. *Hands and Hearts: A History of Court-ship in America.* New York: Basic Books, 1984.

Sadovsky, R., Miller, T., Moskowitz, M., and Hackett, G. "Three-year Update of Sildenafil Citrate (Viagra) Efficacy and Safety." *International Journal of Clini-cal Pharmacology* 55: 115–128, 2001.

Schiavi, Raul C. *Aging and Male Sexuality.* Cambridge: Cambridge University Press, 1999.

Schover, Leslie. *Sexuality and Cancer: For the Woman Who Has Cancer and Her Partner, and Sexuality and Can-cer: For the Man Who Has Cancer and His Partner,* American Cancer Society, 2001.

———., and Soreu Jensen. *Sexuality and Chronic Illness: A Comprehensive Approach.* New York: Guilford, 1988.

Sipski, Marca L., and Craig J. Alexander (Eds). *Sexual Function in People with Disability and Chronic Ill-ness: A Health Professional's Guide.* Gaithersburg, MD: Aspen Publishers, 1997.

Starr, Bernard D., and Marcella B. Weiner. *The Starr-Weiner Report on Sex and Sexuality in the Mature Years.* Briarcliff Manor, NY: Stein and Day, 1981.

Utian, Wolf, and Ruth Jacobowitz. *Managing Your Meno-pause.* New York: Prentice-Hall, 1990.

Walsh, Patrick C. *The Prostate: A Guide for Men and the Women Who Love Them.* New York: New York: Warner Books, 1997.

————. Walsh's Guide to Surviving Prostate Cancer. New York: Warner Books, 2001.

Whitehead, E., Douglas and Terry Malloy. *Viagra: The Wonder Drug for Peak Performance.* New York: Dell Publishing, 1999.

Wolfe, Daniel. *Men Like Us: The GMHC Complete Guide to Gay Men's Sexual, Physical, and Emotional Well-Being.* New York: Ballantine Books, 2000.

Zilbergeld, Bernard. *The New Male Sexuality: The Truth About Men, Sex, and Pleasure.* New York: Bantam, 1993.

INDEX

Reach to Recovery program
(American Cancer
Society), 164
rectum, 87
Reingold, Jacob, 241–42
relationships, finding new,
253–82
activities for, 255–65
adult children and, 279–
80
etiquette for, 254–55
exploitation and, 267–68
handling refusals, rebuffs,
and disappointments,
277–78
issues for men, 270–71
issues for women, 268–70
for lesbian, gay, bisexual,
or transgender (LGBT)
persons, 272–76
living together unmarried,
281–82
qualities for fostering,
265–66
qualities that hinder,
266–67
sexual involvement and,
276–77, 278–79
relaxation therapies, 50
religious activities, 257
Remeron, 146
renal disease, 89–90
research data, 2

*Resource Guide: Lesbian and
Gay Aging*, 274
*Resource Guide of Continence
Products and Services*,
86
rest, 204–7
retirement, 235–36
retropubic (or suprapubic)
surgery, 171–72
reunions, 261–63
revascularization, 135–36
rheumatoid arthritis, 77–78,
80
Ritalin, 147
romance, 329–30
Roosevelt, Eleanor, 332

*Safer Sex Condom Guide for
Men and Women, The*,
96
SAGE News & Events, 274
SAGE (Senior Action in the
Gay Environment),
274
saline implants, 163
sarcopenia, 202
Schover, Leslie R., 76
Schutzler, Michael, 262
second language of sex,
331–32, 333–35
selective estrogen receptor
modulators (SERMs),
43

ABOUT THE AUTHORS

ROBERT N. BUTLER, M.D.

Dr. Robert N. Butler, a Pulitzer Prize winner, has been Brookdale Professor and chairman of the Department of Geriatrics and Adult Development of Mount Sinai Medical Center in New York City from 1982 to 1995. He is now president and CEO of the International Longevity Center-USA, New York City. He is a graduate of Columbia College and the Columbia University College of Physicians and Surgeons.

As chairman of the first Department of Geriatrics in an American medical school, Dr. Butler is a national leader in improving the quality of life for older people. He came to Mount Sinai from the National Institutes of Health, where he was the founding director of the National Institute on Aging in 1976 and served as its first director. Under his leadership, the need for federal funding for research in gerontology gained recognition. One of his achievements was the establishment of research programs for the study of Alzheimer's disease.

A prolific writer, he won the Pulitzer Prize in 1976 for his book *Why Survive? Being Old in America.* He is a member of the Institute of Medicine of the National Academy of Sciences, a founding Fellow of the American Geriatrics Society, and has served as a consultant to the United States Senate Special Committee on Aging, the National Institute of Mental Health, Commonwealth Fund, the Donald W. Reynolds Foundation, and numerous other organizations. He has served as editor-in-chief of the journal *Geriatrics.*

MYRNA I. LEWIS, PH.D.

Dr. Myrna I. Lewis is a psychotherapist, social worker, gerontologist, and writer with a special interest in the social and health issues of midlife and older women. She is an assistant clinical professor at the Mount Sinai School of Medicine in New York City (Department of Community and Preventive Medicine). She maintains a private psychotherapy practice and received her doctorate in social work at Columbia University. She is a fellow of the New York Academy of Medicine.

Dr. Lewis has coauthored a book with Dr. Robert Butler and Dr. Trey Sunderland, *Aging and Mental Health: Positive Psychosocial and Biomedical Approaches* and, with Dr. Robert Butler, *Midlife Love Life,* as well as numerous articles in professional and popular publications. For seven years Dr. Lewis wrote a monthly psychology column entitled "Feelings," for *New Choices Magazine (Readers Digest)* for the age group fifty to seventy. She makes frequent appearances on radio and TV on the subjects of aging and on women's issues as well as lecturing to professional and public groups in the United States and internationally. She is a member of the United Nations' Nongovernmental Committee on Aging and serves on the journal editorial boards of *Clinical Gerontologist* and *Gerontology and Geriatric Education.* She is also a member of corporate advisory boards related to aging.